CAST

TO BE

CHIROPRACTORS

Dr. Liam P. Schübel

Dr. Judd Nogrady

Cast To Be Chiropractors

First printing 2012
Hardcover edition

ISBN 10: 0615556108
ISBN 13: 978-0-615-55610-9

Artwork by Mike Jaroszko

Editing, cover and book design by David Fosbenner

July 1, 2012
Edinburgh Lectures
Scotland

Palmer Family!
Let's take over the
world with TIC!

"The bigger the vision the bigger the life."

-Dr. Liam Schübel, Chiropractor

ADIO y ADIOS,

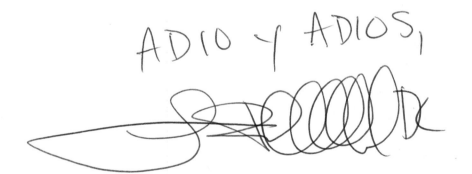

What people are saying about

CAST TO BE CHIROPRACTORS...

I loved *Cast to be Chiropractors*. A fun and interesting book which needs to be read by every chiropractor worldwide. It encourages readers to relive their own journey of finding what chiropractic is to them, and brings back memories of getting the Big Idea for the first time.

I was able to experience Liam and Judd's passion and growth while they traveled down their own road to success, and so will every reader who picks this wonderful book up.

-Outlaw Jim Dubel
www.nbchiro.com

"I loved the book. It was written with great style and humor and illustrates the journeys of two different chiropractors. My journey was totally different, which is why I enjoyed the book so much."

-Reggie Gold
www.reggiegold.com

"Not since Fred Barge's "life without fear" have I been moved like this. *Cast to be Chiropractors* is a profound reminder of the power and enormity of chiropractic."

-Dr. Angus Pyke
2011 Australian Chiropractor of the Year

Cast to be Chiropractors is an exciting read. Dr. Liam and Dr. Judd take us on an extraordinary journey as they grow and develop their passion for chiropractic. This book will inspire you to push past your boundaries and ignite your passion to serve humanity."
-Thom Gelardi, D. C.
Founder, Sherman College of Straight Chiropractic

"Join these chiropractic visionaries as they share their journey to inspire others in the book *Cast to be Chiropractors*. Dr. Liam Schubel and Dr. Judd Nogrady tell their story in this heartfelt and engaging book. See how any person can, must, and will change the world. Enjoy the book, and the journey."
-Christopher Kent, DC, JD
www.subluxation.com

"I love to hear stories of journeys, especially chiropractic ones. Here are two friends with one calling. Two styles but still one profession. Most importantly, two personalities focused on one objective.

Enjoy this read, think about your own journey, amp up, there are people to serve and only the chiropractor contributes to removing interference with mental impulses. Thanks for sharing this Liam and Judd."
-Bill Decken, DC, ACP
Chair, Philosophy Department
Sherman College of Chiropractic
www.sherman.edu

"If you ever wondered where the source of inspiration is for a chiropractor, this book is the map that will show you the way. Drs. Schubel and Nogrady masterfully share from the heart their chiropractic story and invite the reader to do the same. This book is a must read for chiropractors and chiropractic students."

-Eric G. Russell, DC, DPhCS
President, New Zealand College of Chiropractic
www.chiropractic.ac.nz

―――――――――――――――

"What a gift! Thank you Dr. Schubel and Dr. Nogrady for capturing our calling as chiropractors. This is the perfect gift for every chiropractor I know."

-Dr. Shane Walker, President
International Federation of
Chiropractors and Organizations
www.ifcochiro.org

―――――――――――――――

"Once you pick up this book you will not want to put it down. The life experiences and chiropractic journeys shared are touching and motivating, whether you are a chiropractor or not."

-Dr. Nicholas Necak
President, Peruvian Chiropractic Alliance
www.pca.com.pe

"I just landed in New Zealand , and read *Cast to be Chiropractors* overnight on the plane. Wow! I couldn't put it down and can't wait for the second volume. Drs. Schubel and Nogrady are the epitome of loving service and dedication to chiropractic.

This book represents a global vision for chiropractic and is a must read for those looking to make the world a better place. I recommend this book to anyone who wants to walk alongside two powerful, significant chiropractors living their dream of spreading the gift of chiropractic to humanity."
-Dr Brian D. Kelly, President
Life Chiropractic College West
www.lifewest.edu

———————————————————

"This is the book you wish you'd read when you started out in life! Both Judd Nogrady and Liam Schubel give a remarkably refreshing, honest and intimate account of their enduring love of chiropractic. From the very outset, their unyielding passion and purpose hits fast and hits good.

I defy anyone to read it and not be inspired to dig even deeper to share chiropractic with humanity. A superb read that's hard to put down!"
-Maired Howe Rothman
Editor of Spizz Magazine
www.spizzmagazine.com

"Perseverance. Boldness. Bravery. Belief. Determination. Words every great leader and person need to own. Success in chiropractic is about staying true to your principles and vision in the face of challenge, and leading your patients to their health goals.

Drs. Liam and Judd show that you can't be great in one area of your life and mediocre in another if you wish to lead and have impact. With this book, these leaders in our profession light the path for us to follow."

-Ross McDonald, DC
President, Scottish Chiropractic Association
Founder/Owner, The Edinburgh Lectures
www.chiropracticlectures.com

"*Cast to be Chiropractors* is a great, easy read on the lighter side. It's the journey of two chiropractic leaders on their paths towards a life full of purpose through chiropractic. This book will entertain you, make you laugh, but most of all, it will remind you how amazing it is to be a chiropractor, to love and take care of humanity."

-Billy DeMoss DC
Founder and Frontman, Cal Jam
www.californiajam.org

Table of Contents

Acknowledgements

"We stand on the shoulders of Giants."

I would like to thank the following people who have been instrumental to inspiring my personal and professional development. There are many others that I have not named for questions of space and faulty memory but I thank them as well.

My loving wife Parinda, my son Liam Jr., my daughter Maryanne, my parents William Felix Schübel Jr. and Marie Schübel.

My brothers: Dr. Brian Schübel, Brendan Schübel, and Colin Schübel, my uncle Seamus Kerrigan, my grandfather William Felix Schübel Sr.

Dr. J.T Kwon, Dr. David A. Rogosky, Dr. D.D. Palmer, Dr. B.J. Palmer, Dr. Sid Williams, Dr. Thom Gelardi, Dr. Reggie Gold, Dr. Fred Barge, Dr. Jim Dubel, Dr. Joe Strauss, Dr. Christopher Kent, Dr. Brian Kelly, Dr. Ross McDonald, Dr. Michael Sontheimer, Dr. Christopher Taylor, Dr. Bradley Rauch, Dr. Peter Morgan, Dr. Nick Necak, Dr. Emily Broniak, Dr. Richard J. Santo, Dr. Walter Sanchez, Dr. Raymond Page, Dr. Myron Brown, Dr. Adam Nogrady, Dr. Judd Nogrady, Dr. Terry Rondberg, Cinthya Cardenas, Julinho Cardenas, Luis Davila, Ana Avalos, Pedro Paredes, Naydu Paredes, Alba Avalos, and Don Fernando Avalos.

-Dr. Liam Schübel

I would like to thank my family for their continued patience and trust.

Dr. Veronica Nogrady, Dr. Adam Nogrady, Dr. Jill Nogrady, Dr. Alec Nogrady and my children Montana and Jacob.

Most importantly I would like to honor the one person responsible for all our success, my grandfather David Brock. My grandfather never passed five years of formal education yet his knowledge on the world was expansive. His thirst for life was unquenchable and his energy was unmatchable. He lived life at its fullest until his death at 88 years of age. In all the years I was privileged to know him I never heard him utter a discourteous word about anyone, and his one maxim "Succeed not for yourself, but so that the next guy who comes along can have it a little easier" is a way of life that can benefit all mankind. It is in his memory that we all achieve and try to make the world a better place for the "next guy."

All my love and respect,

-Dr. Judd Nogrady

Preface

During the creation of this book I was constantly asked, "What's it going to be about?" The answer "chiropractic" never seemed to be enough for most people. This book was written so that you would stand up and take notice that chiropractic is under attack.

The enemies are at the front gate and at the back door. The enemies of chiropractic are from within and without. We are literally surrounded. Many within the profession have preached peace. There can be no peace with this enemy; they will stop at nothing short of complete annihilation of chiropractic and everything we stand for.

Chiropractors are by nature tough but gentle souls full of life energy. We are protectors of the power that animates the world. We are "life bringers." We recognize that we do not do the healing, but instead remove interference so that the body may function at its best. It is difficult for many of us to get and stay angry because it is not in our nature to do so. I am asking you to get past angry. *I am asking you to take action.*

This is our opportunity to help chiropractic remain pure. This is our chance to let chiropractic be practiced for generations to come. If we don't stand up, no one else will.

Some may ask "What is the problem?" The problem is that if you believe what I believe, then you, like me, are in danger of becoming extinct. Specifically, I believe that:

- The vertebral subluxation damages all aspects of health.

- Every man, woman, and child should be checked and adjusted if necessary by a chiropractor.

- Every newborn should have their upper cervical area checked and adjusted if necessary, within hours after birth. Within minutes if possible.

- The chiropractic adjustment has a pre- and post-analysis that is independent of how a person feels.

- People should have the freedom not to use drugs if they choose.

- Chiropractic should be separate and distinct from the practice of medicine.

- Chiropractic colleges should teach the science, art, and philosophy of chiropractic as their main focus.

- Every student in a chiropractic college should be taught to analyze the spine for subluxation using the recognized technique of their choice.

We need committed individuals to band together and help form a strong alliance to save chiropractic. If we don't, then chiropractic is dead.

Some tell me that I am too late. They say that chiropractic as we know it has reached its last breath. I prefer to think and act like a famous Chechen rebel who, while facing insurmountable odds against a Soviet aggressor, was asked, "How can you win? You have no weapons. You have no food. What will you do?" His reply was chilling. "We will throw rocks and eat Russians." We must adopt this attitude. Are you willing to fight for the principle of chiropractic? I am. I will stand up. I will be heard. I will tell the world that pure chiropractic must survive!

The people are clamoring for our type of care. We need to stand up and deliver the message. Read our story and reignite your passion to serve the world with chiropractic.

A word of explanation

We have not attempted in this book to write an autobiography. This is not our story – it's the story of chiropractic. This story is an attempt to share our view on the greatest healing art the world has ever known. It is homage to the great men and women that have practiced the healing art of chiropractic. To try and make a list of which chiropractors have made the greatest impact would be fruitless as we have been blessed with an abundance of strong personalities that have given much to our profession.

Today there is an infinite amount of talk about what direction we should head. It's easy to forget that just a few short years ago chiropractors risked imprisonment and financial ruin simply by showing up at the office and practicing chiropractic. These strong minded, independent individuals routinely practiced forty years or more doing what they loved. We've been fortunate to rub shoulders with some of these early practitioners. Their history is our history. Their faith and legacy has become ours.

Our sincerest desire is for you to share chiropractic with all of humanity. We hope you come to the same realization that we have, that the only way to achieve your own happiness is to help others live happy, healthy and productive lives. This is the most noble path we know.

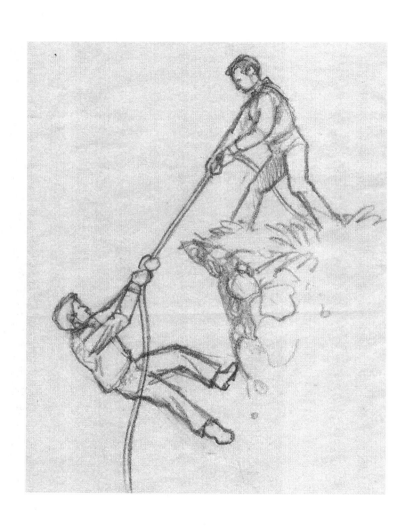

CHAPTER 1

Friends forever

Dr. Judd Nogrady

Becoming a chiropractor has become a popular career choice. Until recently, we chiropractors were chosen by a higher power. It was usually through an accident or sickness. One by one we were rescued through the miracle of chiropractic. We regained our health and our lives, and were reborn with a new dedication to a unique and revolutionary health service called chiropractic. Collectively we were pulled from the fire of ill-health and given the gift of that something extra. We were cast to be chiropractors.

Chiropractic is not a career choice, it's a life choice. It's a life fought uphill, without letup. Chiropractic is about a few rugged individuals committed to helping others. The goal of this book is to help other chiropractors see the tremendous responsibility they have to the people of the world. We must ensure that the greatest discovery in healing is kept sacred and, most importantly, that it is shared with all humanity.

By chance, Dr. Liam Schübel and I met at chiropractic college. We were study partners who became lifelong friends. One of the things everyone needs in order to live the best life possible is a good friend. We chose to write this book together because we want chiropractors and lay people alike to live the life they deserve.

Dr. Liam and I are very different in many ways. Most people know Dr. Liam as an American-born chiropractor who's an inspiration to the entire profession. He's an educator to millions who lectures worldwide.

I've chosen a very different path. I have a home practice as well as three office locations, in New York City and upstate New York. I rarely travel. I seldom see other professionals unless I'm adjusting them at my home office. Some would say I live in my own world. But what I do with all of my being is help others realize their full potential with the chiropractic adjustment.

One of my favorite parts of chiropractic is the house calls I do two days per week. Being able to provide newborns and their mothers with care is vitally important. I spend my days and nights adjusting families, rarely getting out of my routine.

Dr. Liam and I live worlds apart, but we share the same love and deep compassion for chiropractic and our fellow chiropractors. This book is designed to help others achieve a life filled with love, abundance, and a deep, meaningful purpose.

We want you to have a friend in chiropractic. A friend to help you share your dreams, a friend to help you up when you slip, a friend to push you on when you stop or slow down, but most importantly, a friend who, like you, shares a passion for the most remarkable profession in the world, chiropractic.

Liam P. Schübel, DC

When my lifelong friend Dr. Judd Nogrady and I began discussing this book, I must say the idea didn't appeal to me at first. I'm primarily a movement guy, and the idea of sitting in front of a computer typing didn't appeal to me. However, the more we discussed the idea of a book, the more I realized how much we both could share with others.

Dr. Judd is a solid, dependable, rock of a chiropractor. He can always be counted on to give his unvarnished opinion. He leads an exemplary life of deep commitment to his family, friends, and chiropractic. Dr. Judd is one of the few people I know who's not only embraced chiropractic, but completely interwoven it within himself. Many chiropractors, including myself, have been fortunate to share his complete commitment to our art. During the twenty years I've been privileged to know Dr. Judd, I've never known him to waver from his family, chiropractic, or our friendship.

My own deep love for our profession has me living life in what I call organized chaos. I divide my time between running multiple offices in Peru and the Dominican Republic, coaching chiropractors to be successful, managing a chiropractic seminar and products business, promoting chiropractic mission trips, being politically active in the International Federation of Chiropractors and Organizations (IFCO), and participating as an active member on the Board of Trustees for Sherman College of Chiropractic in South Carolina, USA. My life is completed at home, as a father to my two beautiful children, Liam Jr. and Maryanne, and a husband to my loving wife, Parinda.

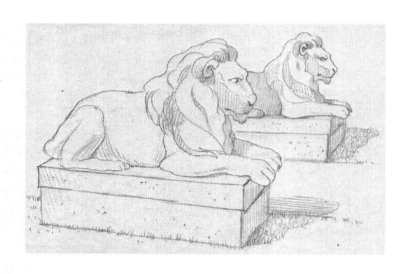

CHAPTER 2

A path set in stone

Judd

Living life with a deep commitment to chiropractic is not an easy path. You must lead rather then follow. You must put others in front of yourself. It means rarely having a normal dinner or bed time. It means total commitment to others and to the art, "your art," of chiropractic.

Most people don't choose a life path for themselves. Instead, they live their years letting life just happen to them. They rarely look up or side- to-side. They just take what comes along and pass on without a ripple. Others, however, make choices, goals, and long term plans. They usually live longer, more fulfilling lives and are productive for all of their years.

Then there are still others who are chosen through no decision of their own. The universe reaches out and plucks them from the multitudes, setting them toward a specific path. They don't worry what others think, and they couldn't care less about the platitudes of the masses. They're too busy serving others. When they pass, a huge hole in the fabric of life is altered until another is chosen to fill the void. They are chiropractors, and if you are one or are planning on being one, you have huge shoes to fill and a universe to serve.

Chiropractors of a few generations ago routinely practiced for *forty years or more*. They never wavered off course. They were masters at promoting life and relieving human suffering. They always had time to talk about their faith, and they always made time for one more adjustment. When I was chosen to be a chiropractor a very stubborn practitioner must have just left!

I was a twenty year old New York City police officer with a scrap metal business on the side. Work was easy for me. All things were accomplished with brute force. When in doubt, use more force. Any problem I ever had could always be solved with force. My philosophy was "when in doubt, hit it harder." Is the suspect resisting arrest? Hit him harder! Is the metal too long to fit in the truck? Get a sledge hammer and hit it harder! Does someone disagree with you? Hit them harder! It was a simple way to live life, but when my wakeup call came, life hit *me* harder so I would take notice.

I'd been hauling scrap metal and garbage in and around New York City since I was sixteen years old. I bought my first truck before I even had a license. I routinely missed school for work, and never ever had any thought of doing anything else. I only went to school on Mondays and Fridays. The reason I attended at all was to get a diploma to satisfy my very tough, but not too strict mother.

I became a police officer almost by accident. A friend of mine desperately wanted to become an officer. He asked me to drive him to the exam center, because I was the only one that he knew with a reliable vehicle. When we arrived at the testing center, they had an option of taking the test as a walk-in. Rather than hanging around, I went in and took the test. I passed the exam, and within six months, was called to begin my police training.

At that time, the New York City police academy was noted for having the best police education in the world. After graduation I was assigned to solo foot patrol in Bedford-Stuyvesant, Brooklyn, New York, 73rd precinct. This precinct is noted as being in one of the worst neighborhoods in New York City.

Next I rotated between the 73rd, 75th, 77th, and 82nd precincts, considered to be some of the most violent neighborhoods in the United States. As a police officer in these areas my hit it harder philosophy worked extremely well.

At twenty years old my friends and family thought that I had it all. My junk business was booming. My police career provided the long term security of life insurance, health insurance, and a twenty year pension allowing me to retire at forty. I would be a fool to quit. That's what "everyone" said. Yet with just one year down and nineteen to go, the more I did police work, the less I liked it. With that on my mind, I did what almost no cop ever does: I quit. This is so unusual in the police business that my sergeant, in his twenty-nine years of experience, had never done the paperwork on anyone who'd quit so suddenly.

The final procedures involved the surrender of my weapon, an exit interview, and a few shakes of the stunned sergeant's head. When I made that decision to walk out, I showed the universe I was someone who could be counted on to do what I thought was right. I am convinced that chiropractic called me that day. However, she knew it would take a hard hit to get me on the proper path.

People always ask why I quit the police department. The job of a police officer is an excellent career choice for many people. However, where I worked, it felt like a life without purpose. I was writing tickets to fill quotas, and arresting people only to see them back out on the street the next day. It all seemed to be a pointless exercise in futility.

My scrap metal business, by contrast, was easy to understand. The work could be long, hard, and heavy, but you were paid by weight. The harder you worked, the more money you made. There were issues, but none that couldn't be worked out with your fists or by hard work.

Another benefit of lifting heavy metal all day is a great body with big muscles, something my wife never lets me forget. I have no doubt that I'd still be hauling scrap metal today if not for a small, but life-changing slip. As it turned out, chiropractic called me with an injury.

One day on a job, two employees and I were carrying an old, extremely heavy cast iron bathtub down a flight of steep stairs in ninety degree heat. I was holding the tub with both hands while walking backwards, while the two other men were holding the other end. I took the first step down a long multilevel staircase, but before my foot reached the second step, someone had a small slip. That small slip changed who I was forever.

We lost control of the tub and I took a long ride, tub on top, all the way down the stairs. It would've been bad enough to fall down this long, hard, steep, flight of stairs, but I fell down with an over 300 pound tub on top of me!

When I regained consciousness I was lying face down. Everything hurt, and I mean everything! One of my employees quickly came to my aid and the two of us pushed and pulled the tub off of me. When the second man came over to help, he took one look and threw up on me. I knew then that it must be bad. I was bleeding from a number of wounds, and there were lacerations and blunt force trauma all over my body. When I tried but was unable to stand, I knew I was badly injured. For the first time in my life my body let me down, and my philosophy of "hit it harder" failed.

I'd been injured at work before. I'd endured multiple concussions and numerous minor injuries, but nothing like this. I crawled to my truck and drove myself to the hospital.

My first experience with the medical profession started out well. I was hurt, and they were there to help me. I'd like to point out that there are many loving, caring, truly honest people in the medical profession. The problem is they just don't have the required education to be truly effective. I won't go through the various tests, specialists and poor diagnosis and prognosis that I received. The end medical conclusion was that I was disabled "forever." I was faced with a lifetime of poor health and no chance of working again.

Liam

As I write this chapter I am 40,000 feet in the air headed to the Dominican Republic to help promote chiropractic. Expanding the vision and reach of chiropractic throughout the world is my passion. Helping to spread the life restoring gift of chiropractic with other dedicated, passionate, loving, subluxation-centered chiropractors is my vision.

Dr. D.D. Palmer is officially recognized as the discoverer of chiropractic. His son Dr. B.J Palmer was considered the developer of chiropractic. One of my great mentors, Dr. Sid Williams, has been called "the defender of chiropractic." Where do I fit in? I believe I've been called to be "chiropractic's ambassador to the world." My vision and life's work is centered on nothing else.

While traveling to the most remote corners of the world, I've witnessed some of the most amazing results of chiropractic care. The world's populations have been looking for exactly what chiropractic delivers. Chiropractic care gives them the chance to live life at its greatest potential.

My passion in chiropractic started back in Freehold, New Jersey, USA, with the most loving person I know: my mom. When I was growing up, my mom had always been there for my three brothers and myself. Looking back, I think she must be one of the most loving people I've ever known. She always made sure our family was loved, fed and safe.

When mom began to have pain in both her shoulders we were very concerned. When it became debilitating, life became unbearable for her. She decided to seek help. Her first course of action was to go to the family medical doctor. He did an examination and prescribed medication. The drugs didn't help though, and her symptoms became worse and worse.

In addition, the side effects on my mother's stomach and mood were too much for her to bear. Several more trips to the medic provided similarly miserable results, and always more medications. At a friend's urging, my mom went to see a chiropractor. The results were nothing short of miraculous!

This is when the seed of chiropractic was planted in my life. Chiropractic care helped the person that mattered most in my life. Very few people on this earth have the blessing to be passionate about their life's work. In my experience, that passion comes from discovering one's purpose in life, and working to fulfill it.

One of my hero's, Dr. Sid Williams, used to say, "There is nothing sadder than a young person without a purpose." Youth is the time when we're all scrambling to understand the meaning and changes in our lives. Who are we? Why are we here? What are we going to do with the rest of our lives? Some extremely fortunate people know from a very young age exactly what their life's work is going to be. Others struggle to find themselves, and some spend a lifetime looking for that one thing that will give them true satisfaction and fulfillment.

From a very early age I can remember praying to God for guidance. I felt I had a very close and personal relationship with Him. I can vividly recall taking every opportunity to ask for His guidance with my life and future plans.

From my earliest memories in childhood, I always felt that my life had meaning, and that I was destined to help others. I knew that somehow my purpose in life was to help others in some way. I just didn't know how.

Growing up, many of my classmates came from neighborhoods with large houses, expensive cars, the nicest clothes, and the coolest sneakers. Boy do I remember the sneakers! Fancy sneakers were the ultimate symbol of being cool when I was young.

Going shopping with my mom for school clothes every year was a humbling experience. I'm eternally grateful that my parents earned enough money to buy us new school clothes, but in a world of bullies and "cool guys," my humble collection of clothing put me on the bottom of the "cool guy" list.

My dad believed that haircuts were something that was every father's responsibility. Although he was a great dad, he was a poor barber. He left little hair and seemed to take delight in accentuating the size of my ears with his old fashioned sheep shears.

Every year I remember wishing I could disappear during the first roll call. The teacher would read down the list, and mispronounce my name as Lie Am, which everyone would laugh at. It felt like every eye was on me, and boy did I stick out with my value-oriented clothes, bargain sneakers and very personal style of haircut. Now, however, I realize that not being part of the "in crowd" is valuable experience for being a chiropractor.

What I lacked in coolness, I made up in the grades department. I always did well in school. Not because I was the smartest in the class, but because I never gave up. I kept trying until I mastered each lesson. That dogged persistence has made all the difference in my life. In spite of some challenging school experiences, my self-esteem would not be shaken. I knew that no matter what, I could do it. I had this inner voice telling me to never give up, because one day I'd help others in ways I could only dream about.

I was a good student throughout grade and middle school. In my junior year of high school I was close to being a straight A student. I knew I had to go to college, but nothing really seemed to hold my interest. With time running out, I decided to further my studies in the subject I did best in, computer science! I chose Trenton State College in New Jersey to study computer science because it was considered one of the best public colleges in the United States.

My dad was happy because being a New Jersey resident entitled me to a reduced tuition. I remember the bill for the first year was six thousand dollars. I was absolutely amazed that school could cost so much money! My dad made it absolutely clear that he expected great things from me for his six thousand dollars.

I packed up my things and got ready to move out on my own for the first time in my life. The college was only forty-five minutes from home. I packed everything I needed into my 1981 Chevy Chevette hatchback. My mom was nervous about me moving out, but she was happy that the school was relatively close by. With hugs and kisses from my mom and handshakes from my dad, I was off at the maximum speed the Chevette would go, a whopping fifty miles per hour down the New Jersey Turnpike!

For those of you not familiar with cars, the Chevy Chevette is at the absolute opposite end of the spectrum from the Chevy Corvette. It was mustard yellow with rusted out floors and a large dent in the driver's door. The transmission was a standard four speed, with no reverse! Nothing's more humiliating then having to push your car backward from a parking space. Let's just say it definitely *didn't* attract the girls.

As with many of the other new students, it didn't take me long to abuse my new found freedom. My excellent study habits slipped drastically and I learned how to party. Like everything else in my life, I did it to the maximum. I quickly found out that computers were not my thing. I loved people. I found myself sitting in a classroom with students whose best friend was their computer! I have no idea how I pulled out straight D's in my first semester. The only thing I learned was where to get cheap pizza and beer.

Needless to say, my parents were extremely disappointed with me. My dad let me know this in no uncertain terms as soon as I arrived home for summer break. Dad laid it on the line. I had one more semester to improve, or his money and I weren't going back to Trenton State. He also made it clear that if I wasn't in school, I'd be getting a job. I must admit that, at the time, going to work sounded much better than going back to college.

During the break, I looked into the jobs available for the skills I had. It was a quick, sobering experience. It didn't take long to realize that college was a better decision. I decided to go back with a new purpose. My first decision was to get out of computer science! I needed to pick a new major, quick. I asked myself what do I like doing best? Well, other than partying, it was hanging out with my new friends. Most of them were majoring in communications.

My friends were fun, vibrant, and excited about what they were doing. They were a unique group of individuals who I enjoyed being around. I felt a common bond with other people enjoying life. I decided I was going to have a career in radio or television, and my new major would help me achieve my goals.

The first course I took was Radio Production, taught by Dr. David Rogosky. It changed my life. Everyone called him "Dr. Dave." Dave was a character. His three constants were body movement, a cigar in his mouth, and a cup of coffee in his hand. Dave was always professional in his actions and his attire. Those who got to know him well found that he had a genius mind and liked to have fun.

Dave was a communications visionary. He told us how someday analogue television and radio would be a thing of the past. Some day we would have digital high definition television. In the late 1980's, we thought he was crazy. It all seemed so complicated, and prohibitively expensive. I only wish I'd bought stock in everything he told us about.

Looking back at his bold predictions, it was as if he could see the future.

Dr. Dave came from a small oil town in Pennsylvania. His dad was a Pennsylvania state trooper. Dave had learned that education provided multiple opportunities to a more promising and fulfilling life. He earned his doctorate degree in communications and quickly applied for a teaching position. As a professor, he had great benefits, a relaxing lifestyle, and summers off. I spent many summers with him learning about his other passion, boating.

One summer we rented a forty foot trawler. Dave had his captain's license, and it was a beautiful boat. That summer was one of the best I've ever had. We went from town to town along the Chesapeake Bay enjoying the ocean, smoking cigars, drinking beer, and fishing.

While Dr. Dave taught me many things, the most important was how to speak with authority. One night a storm blew up. The rain and fog rolled in, and the boat felt as if it would split as ten foot waves crashed over the bow. I was beyond nervous, so I asked Dave if everything was okay. He replied calmly, almost humorously, that this storm was "just a little blow" and that he had been through much worse.

He spent all night at the wheel while I helped by reading charts and manning the bilge pump. The next morning I asked Dave to tell me about the other big storms that he'd been through. He burst out laughing, and told me he thought we were going to die. It'd been the worst storm by far that he'd ever seen! He knew, however, that if he told me the truth, I might not have been able to help him as calmly and effectively as I did. He truly was the master of the situation.

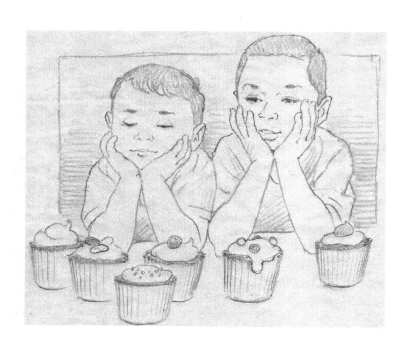

CHAPTER 3

Decisions, decisions, decisions

Judd

I'd love to write that the next step was that I went to a chiropractor, got adjusted, and got well. Case closed! Hurray for chiropractic! The truth is a little stickier. I did go to a chiropractor. He was attentive, professional, and very thorough. He reviewed all my medical tests and even took some more X-rays. He told me my case was very difficult, and told me to come back on Friday for a report of findings. Wow! I was impressed he was going to spend a whole day going over my case!

Well, when Friday came, I limped in and received my report of findings. Honestly, I don't remember a word he said, but it was an impressive report full of charts marked with red ink, long term goals, and color photos. It sounded great! I was eager to begin.

I was led to a "treatment room" and hooked to an electric machine. After about fifteen minutes they unhooked me and I could barely move. I limped out to the front desk and received a bill equal to any doctor up to that point. To say I had my doubts about this new care would be an understatement, but I stuck with it every other day for three weeks. During the course of "the treatment" I was put on different machines all with the same outcome: misery.

Next I had a follow up visit with the chiropractor. He recommended more "treatments," but he indicated that he wasn't quite sure what my outcome would be. I went out to my truck and slumped down in the front seat. I was truly out of hope. I am not a religious man, but I did what was probably the most sensible thing that I had done up to this point: I prayed. I spent a good amount of time at it. I promised that if I got help, I would do something useful with my life. I just wanted an answer and some relief. I drove off, feeling silly for trying to make deals with the universe.

I had six dollars left in my pocket, so I decided to go to the deli and get some lunch. I ordered bologna on a bagel with mayo and mustard, tomato and onion. While I was waiting, the man next to me struck up a conversation. He saw how I limped and how bad I looked, so he gave me the name of his chiropractor. I almost laughed! I told him I just left the chiropractor, and I'd been to every M.D. available. He wouldn't take No for an answer. He told me "Don't worry, my chiropractor is different!" Had I been healthier and stronger, I may have hit him, but I was desperate!

He kept saying "my chiropractor." He was emphatic that "his chiropractor" could help me. Finally I relented, and this guy actually led me to his chiropractor's office.

When we arrived there, it was just a house with a one word sign, "Chiropractor." I noticed there were many cars parked in front, but the place looked so unlike any office I'd been to before. There was a cat lying out in the sun next to the front door. There were kids' toys lying on the lawn, and there was a small table outside with people having lunch. It looked like a party or family reunion.

I hesitated at the door, and then thought what the hell, I have nothing to lose. I went in, filled out a very basic form, and then waited for quite a long time in the waiting room. The worn out waiting room, which was decorated with cheap plastic chairs, and an orange carpet from the 1970s, did little to inspire hope.

Yet, as I waited, I noticed families coming in, and by families, I mean mom, dad, and the kids. I began to wonder what I was in for. I thought this was the place for bad backs. I couldn't fathom what all these people were doing here.

Finally my name was called and I was told to wait in room three. As I waited I looked around, but there wasn't much to see, just a few old houseplants, and three chiropractic adjusting tables. One pushed up against a wall, one was standing up (an old Hylo), and the third was what I would learn later was a side posture toggle table.

There was no carpet in this room, just old tile like the kind they used to have in schools. There were three bare spots on the floor, one near each table, which formed a triangle. I remember the three spots because they made me think of the three burned out places that rocket engines leave during a space ship landing in a science fiction movie.

In the middle of the three tables there was a chair that faced the door, and this is where I sat. My file had been left on the outside of the door in a file holder. I heard it pulled out, and then dropped back in. Then the door opened. In walked this old guy, who looked to be at least seventy-five years old.

"Hello," he said. "Please stand on the metal plate."

I got up and stood on the metal plate, which was attached to the bottom of the Hylo adjusting table.

"Reach out and hold the table, then lean forward," he said. Next he said, "The table will lower you down. Please relax."

The table made a noise, and as I was lowered down he asked a few questions. How long did I hurt? What had I done? Was I a student? By the time the table stopped moving, his questions were answered. He put his hands on my spine from T1 to L5 and then pushed a button causing the table to start up again. On the way up he asked a few more questions.

When the table was up, I stepped off the metal plate and onto the floor. The doctor was standing there ready for the next exam. Under his feet was the worn spot on the floor. I started to ask something, but he smiled and held up his hand saying, "Not yet, I have to do a little more checking." All told, I was examined for about three minutes, including the ride up and down.

"Please lay face up on the table," he said, while pointing to the table pushed up against the wall. This time he examined my neck. He placed my head in his palms, and used his fingers to go down through the bones in my neck. Now I'm thinking this guy is nuts, because there's no problem in my neck. Didn't he read the chart?

I start to speak but before I can get the words out he says "OK, stand up." As I stood up, he was standing at the head of the table with his hand grasping a handle on the wall. I looked at his feet and noticed he was standing on another worn out spot on the floor. (Later, I figured out the purpose of the handle was so he could pull himself up after crouching down and checking my neck).

"Almost done son! Now I need you to lie on your side and face the door."

This was the side posture toggle table. I lay down on my side with my head in the little cradle, and he took his position on the last worn out spot on the floor.

I looked into his knees, thinking "What the heck is going on here?" when all of a sudden WHAM, he moved the top bone in my neck! No one ever told this guy that toggle technique was supposed to be gentle! I thought he killed me!

"Now I want you to slowly get up and lay on your back on the table," he said, while pointing to the table against the wall. "Someone will be in to get you in a moment."

Before I could say a word he was gone. I didn't think the old guy could move that fast. I slowly got up and lay back down on the table he directed me to. I started to laugh to myself that this was a "three table exam." I smiled, realizing that it was the first time in a long time that I could smile.

I laid there about five or six minutes until a young lady came in. She smiled and asked how my first adjustment went. I couldn't say a word. I just grinned back at her. Finally she broke the ice.

"I guess you are doing pretty well. The doctor wants you to come to class on Wednesday and schedule an appointment for Friday."

I was in a state of shock feeling like I couldn't do anything but grin. I nodded my head and went out to the front desk. I vaguely heard them set up my class for 10:00 on Wednesday, and appointment for 9:45 on Friday.

I went home, crawled into bed, and slept for fifteen hours without moving a muscle. When I woke up the next day, I knew something was different! I definitely felt better, but more than that, I felt different. Now without going all "hug a tree" in trying to describe this, I realized that for the first time in my life, all the violence was out of me.

To appreciate this, realize that my whole life up until this point had been about body strength and violence. Now I felt completely in love with the world. I walked around in wonder at this new feeling.

When I went to the office for the Wednesday class at 10am, the doctor was there seeing patients. The secretary then informed me that the class was to be held at 10pm! When I went back at 10pm, the same secretary was still there. She had about seven or eight of us go into a classroom in the back of the office, and the doctor came shuffling in.

The doctor explained Chiropractic to us from A to Z. As he went through it all, I noticed how passionate he was, and how much this meant to him. He was so passionate about the material that it felt like he barely noticed us.

As he wrapped up, I glanced at my watch. It was 11:15pm! This guy had been here since 9am. (I later learned that he took a forty-five minute nap every afternoon). That was one heck of a long day for anyone, especially a seventy-five year old plus guy. (I also later learned that he'd been in practice for over forty years, and had actually studied under Dr. B.J. Palmer).

One of the guys in the class with me was there because he'd been in an accident. Numerous steel rods had been surgically placed in his spine. He'd been everywhere and had tried everything. His last surgery made it impossible for him to lie down. He had to sleep in a chair sitting up. Yet through it all, he maintained a good attitude. I immediately stopped feeling sorry for myself, because if he could maintain a positive mindset, so could I.

On my next visit, the doctor laid it all out for me. I was to come twice a week for a while. It was his opinion that the damage to my spine was permanent. However, he felt I'd get some relief, and should be able to start moving again. As I went to leave, he told me to stop at the desk about payment arrangements. Then, just before I walked out, he said, "If you put your mind to it, you'd make a great chiropractor."

At the moment, I didn't think much of that, because I was bracing myself for what I was about to be charged. When I got to the desk, the secretary let me know that I owed $18 for the first exam and adjustment, and another $18 for the second visit. The class was free. My total bill: $36 dollars. I couldn't believe how reasonable it was! After I paid, I began thinking about what the doctor had said about me becoming a chiropractor.

Liam

In college, I was assigned a radio program, which I called "The Screamin' Liam Blues Show." It was classic blues, and it was pure fun playing music that I loved while interacting with callers. Because I was a newer member of the communications department, I wasn't given a choice about my radio time.

In commercial radio, most people will kill for the morning drive spot. Not me! I thrive in the afternoon and late into the evening. I love to sleep in! That's why I scheduled all my classes for the afternoons whenever possible. Unfortunately, the only time spot available for the Screamin' Liam Blues Show was 6am-9am. I take my hat off to the DJ's and talk radio people that can be happy, funny and exciting at 6am. For me, it was pure torture.

I quickly decided that in order to make this radio program work, I'd have to go on the air with someone who was strong in my weak areas, and weak in my strong areas. That combination is what I continue to look for to this day in all my business relationships.

Doug Burroughs was a communications student at Trenton State College. He was on the ten year plan for a four year degree. Not because he wasn't smart, far from it! You see, Doug was legally blind. Cancer had eaten one of his eyes and one of his legs. When I first met Doug, I was horrified. He was shocking to look at. What I found amazing, though, was that over time, as we developed a deep friendship, I no longer noticed his flaws. When I saw him, all I could see was Doug and the amazing person he was.

We were quite a sight going out to the radio program at 5:30am every morning. I lived down the hall from Doug, so I'd walk over and knock on his door when I came to pick him up. He'd grab my shoulder, and I'd be the support for this incredible one legged guy as he'd hop across campus, down to the basement of the student center where the radio station was located.

Doug had an absolutely contagious laugh and a completely goofy sense of humor. In spite of all the adversity in his life, Doug never quit, and he always laughed. Contrasting that, in spite of all my blessings, I was the uptight guy always trying to make our show perfect. Things would inevitably go wrong, and I'd be yelling or screaming, as Screamin' Liam has a tendency to do. Doug would say something funny to show how ridiculous I was acting, and soon the whole crew was laughing along with us. Doug taught me to enjoy the moments that make up the day, and laugh as often and as loud as possible.

Interestingly, our show gained a huge following with the Trenton State Prison population. Though prisoners weren't our intended listeners, we received letter after letter with requests and suggestions for the show. While many inmates made requests, some seemed more like offers we couldn't refuse! Doug and I sometimes complied because it seemed foolish to ignore threats.

During my junior year, as I started to get out into the field with others who were working in real world communications, something became very clear: this was not what I wanted to do with the rest of my life. In the real world, the happy, thriving bunch of people I knew turned into very competitive players, people who would do anything to get ahead.

I also began to ask, what do I want to represent my life's work? A radio or TV show? The thought of spending my life in an artificial world didn't resonate with me. I wanted more. I wanted to make a real difference in people's lives.

I was desperate to find my purpose in life during this time. I'd tried computers and failed, and now I thought I just wasted three years studying a major in electronic communications. If I could've seen what would happen later in my life, I would've known that it was actually an excellent investment in time.

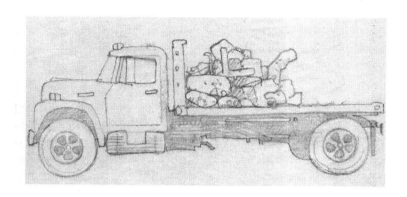

CHAPTER 4

A few bumps in the road

Judd

One of the huge negatives about becoming a chiropractor is that you have to go to college, and for a long time. This is one of the first things I found out when I went to the local library. The next thing is something that's stayed with me. The book said that chiropractors were a few rugged individuals who promulgated the idea that proper alignment of the spine and optimal health are intimately related. Against all odds, chiropractors were gaining acceptance nationally. The book also said that chiropractors should expect to earn about $75,000 a year.

The thing that caught my attention though was "a few rugged individuals." That was it! The old guy was right, I could be a chiropractor! The first thing I had to do was get two years of community college finished with the required prerequisites for chiropractic college. The required classes were Physics I and II, Chemistry I & II, Organic Chemistry I & II, and finally Anatomy I & II. Well, the good thing about never having done any high school work was that I didn't know enough to know that I didn't know enough to pass these classes!

College was a completely new experience for me. I remember sitting through my first lecture watching all the other students writing stuff down. After class, a nice looking girl asked me how I remembered all the information without taking notes. Taking notes? Was that what we were supposed to do? I didn't have a clue. I didn't even bring a notebook or pen!

The first thing I did after class was sign up for after school help. For the next lecture, I had a pen, paper, but still no idea what to do. Luckily for me, after the second lecture I had my extra help session. The tutor was the same person that was teaching the class. She said she never had anyone sign up for extra help on the first day. I explained who I was, what I wanted, and all about chiropractic and my situation.

She looked at me, her eyes getting bigger all the time. Finally she said, "Wait. Stop a minute. You expect to pass college physics, and you've never taken high school math?"

Well, she loved my answer.

"What does physics have to do with math," I asked?

She was so unnerved she just froze for a moment. When she came back to her senses, she held up her hand and told me to wait a minute. She left the room and returned quickly with a practice test, something like an "are you ready for physics?" exam. She placed the exam on the table and said she'd be back in thirty minutes. She instructed me to make sure I did both sides!

I looked at the exam and had no idea what to make of it. I looked so long at the first equation that I remember it to this day. $Y=MX+B$. She came back a half hour later and of course, the test was the same as when she had given it to me, totally blank. I couldn't even begin to fill it out.

She explained slowly and carefully that I would require some basic math before I could hope to pass her class. It was too late for me to switch into basic math, however, and I wasn't willing to do nothing for the whole semester, so I stuck with physics class and failed. I attended every class, and took every test. I had a low score of ten, and my highest score was a fifty, which I got on the final exam. Half correct! I thought I did pretty well!

I wore that poor teacher out by attending every extra help session available. In order for me to get the two year degree with the required prerequisites, I wound up attending Suffolk Community College, Nassau Community College, Orange County Community College, and a few classes at SUNY New Paltz. I was now a seasoned veteran of New York's community colleges. My final prerequisite class was Organic Chemistry, which I'd chosen to take in Atlanta, Georgia, at my chosen chiropractic college.

There are three main lessons I learned about college. First, it's best to go to high school and learn the basics, which is the most cost and time efficient. Second, extra help sessions work in two ways: you get to see all the information twice, and sometimes the teacher gets so sick of seeing you, that they'll pass you just to get you out of their life. Third, when you stick a pipette through your hand on the first day of chemistry lab, people will remember you for a while.

Liam

As a senior year student in communications with no desire to enter that field upon graduation, I returned home to Freehold, New Jersey that summer with the intention of trying to find a profession that would fulfill my true passion in life.

One afternoon my mom asked me to accompany her while she went for her regular chiropractic adjustment. Ever since I was a kid, she'd kept up her weekly regimen of care. I, however, hadn't been adjusted since I was in high school. As soon as I walked in the door, the pleasant memories of my positive childhood experience with chiropractic returned.

The staff was friendly, the atmosphere was lively, and the people were happy. My mom introduced me to her current chiropractor. He told me that chiropractic was about restoring life, and that I, as a chiropractor, could liberate the potential of humanity with a chiropractic adjustment. He was so excited that even after twenty-five years in practice, he couldn't wait to get to the office. This was what I had been looking for, a way to make a positive impact on people's lives. Then and there I made the best decision in my entire life. I decided to become a chiropractor.

My first challenge was how to get a chiropractic education. I soon found out you need the equivalent of two years of basic sciences to be eligible for chiropractic college. After doing all the figuring, I realized that in order to get the classes I would need to enter chiropractic college, it would take two years, but only if I received permission to double up some classes, and exceed the allowable amount of credits per semester. The result was that for my senior year, a time when most students take it easy, I was going to hit the books harder than I ever had before.

These classes weren't going to be easy ones either. I started with Chemistry, Organic Chemistry, Physics and Anatomy. I remember going to visit the Chemistry department head, Dr. Phillip Dumas, and begging him to sign the required paperwork, granting me permission to take the extra classes. Since my grades weren't at the level required to take these extra credit hours, his signature was needed to override the internal college bureaucracy.

I used my new found chiropractic passion to vividly describe my dream of becoming a chiropractor. Thankfully, he saw my commitment and signed off. Years later, after becoming a successful chiropractor and lecturer, I sent him a thank you note. I told him where my life had taken me as a result of his giving me special consideration.

In 1991, I graduated from Trenton State College with a Bachelor's degree in electronic communications. However, it would take an additional year of study to fulfill my chiropractic school's prerequisites. I worked in a bank during the day and went to school at night. Before I knew it, I'd completed my courses, and was ready to start chiropractic college!

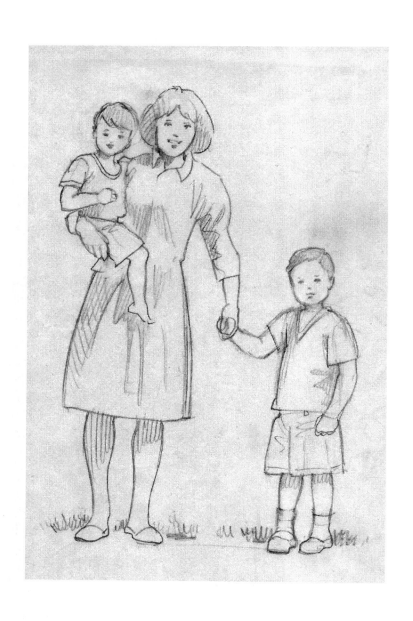

CHAPTER 5

Wide-eyed wonder

Judd

With one prerequisite left, Organic Chemistry (which I'd already taken once and failed miserably), I learned that a chiropractic college in Georgia had a ten week Organic Chemistry class. That is, five weeks for Organic I and five weeks for Organic II. So, of course, I signed up. When I arrived in Georgia for ten weeks of chemistry, it was July, and it was hot! I rented an apartment at the Barclay Arms, which was directly across the street from the college.

My life now consisted of going to class with a pen, paper and a tape recorder, and then going home after class and listening to the recording, while writing down every word the instructor said. I then studied it all again. My life became an uninspiring cycle of study sessions. I became depressed for the first time in my life.

Since I was so close to my goal, it should've been the happiest time in my life. Instead, I was in the greatest depths of despair that I'd ever felt. Why? "Real" work seemed so simple in comparison to constant study. Plus, I was getting fat from too much southern food and too little activity. Finally, having no friends or family around made life extremely lonely.

I hated Georgia. Hot all day, rain every afternoon, and busy all the time. Georgia was pure torture for me. I remember taking my final exam, waiting for the grades to be posted, and then leaving Georgia. As I attempted to leave Atlanta, my truck's air conditioner quit. It was ninety-six degrees out and I was in a humongous traffic jam. I actually said out loud, "I make one promise that whatever I have to do in life, I will never come back to Georgia again." God must like a good laugh, because one year to the day I was in the exact same place, coming back into Atlanta.

I'd been accepted to New York Chiropractic College pending the last prerequisite. I had about four months before chiropractic college officially started. I felt like I'd gone through so much that by now, that graduating was guaranteed.

After graduation, I went home to work with my grandfather on his farm, earn some extra money, and get some fresh air. The first month home was like heaven on earth. It was good to be back in upstate New York. I felt one hundred percent sure that the decision I'd made was the best. New York Chiropractic College had just relocated to beautiful Seneca Falls, and I couldn't wait.

With two months to go, something happened that I was sure never would. I met the girl of my dreams, and fell deeply, and completely, in love. I proposed to Veronica on our first date, and we've been together ever since. Our marriage has been pure happiness.

I left something out, however. In order to marry the girl of my dreams, I had to get past her extremely strict, rigid parents. Her father in particular was a well-respected, revered steel worker. My future father-in-law was one tough guy. Even today when people find out that I married his daughter, they're amazed. He was famous for his unbelievable work ethic, and his marvelously violent temper. Before my first chiropractic adjustment, he was the kind of guy that I'd have taken on head-to-head, win or lose. Now however, the post-adjustment version of me didn't have that mentality anymore.

Time passed until we were about two weeks away from departing for New York Chiropractic College. I was still trying to figure out some way to tell my future father-in-law that we'd be getting married and moving out in about a week or so. I decided to take the direct approach, so I drove over to their house when I knew my fiancé wasn't home. I figured if things went badly, she wouldn't have to see me get beat up, or worse, see me beat up her father!

When I got there I was one nervous guy. I asked my wife's mother if her husband was home. She told me he was out back working on a bulldozer and would welcome some help. When I got out back he was under the machine.

When I got there he asked me to hand him a sledgehammer. Great, I thought, he knows what I want already! While he was pounding on something under the machine, I broke the news to him between whacks.

"Excuse me sir, I know that you know that I have been seeing your daughter a lot."

A grunt and another whack of the hammer was the reply.

"I just wanted to let you know that if it's all right with you, we're going to get married and move out next week."

All grunting and whacking suddenly stopped, and I stood there in the deafening silence. I actually heard him thinking. He slowly came out from under the machine with the sledge hammer in hand. Great! I'm finally going to chiropractic college, and now I'm going to get killed!

His reply was slow in coming.

"What are you planning to do if I say no?"

"Well, we were planning to go anyway, but we really want your consent."

He slowly put down the sledge hammer, which I thought was a step in the right direction. He then gave me this one demand:

"If you want to marry my daughter, you have to buy a house to live in, not rent some place."

I think this was his way of setting an impossible hurdle.

"OK, then I'll buy a house."

The next day I found myself in Port Byron, New York. Port Byron is a small town. I define small town by:

1. How many streets down town has – it had one.

2. If there's a police department – there wasn't.

3. If there's a restaurant – there wasn't.

4. How many stores there are – there was one - Ed and Jean's gas, lotto, wine and deer skinning.

Only in a town like Port Byron could you find a place that we could afford. The house cost $29,000, came with eight acres, and we could move in while the closing was in progress. Yes, we bought a house in one day and moved in within the week!

Love will make you do crazy things, and chiropractic will allow you to keep doing them. We must have been crazy, or just overly optimistic. I include this because every time I hear someone having a little bump in the road on the way to chiropractic college, I think of our many bumps, in fact, so many that it looks like a mogul run on a ski slope. Yet all those supposed bumps turned out to be blessings. All the failures put us into new and fantastic directions. However, the next bump was a big one.

Everything was going great in our new home. It was a short drive to Seneca Falls where I attended college. I even got a job cleaning out horse stalls three mornings a week. I was so excited to attend the first day of orientation that I was two hours early. When I got there, the auditorium was locked, so I waited outside until the custodian arrived and let me in. I was sitting front row and center so I wouldn't miss a thing. Slowly the auditorium filled with sleepy students and faculty. Finally the president of the college arrived, and began his speech.

As he spoke, he described the road for chiropractic as needing to head into a new "more modern medical era." He felt chiropractic would become more accepted only if we were more limited in our approach. He described a new kind of chiropractic that would work hand in hand with medicine. He went on to say that he would personally stamp out any kind of life changing hocus pocus associated with chiropractic.

It started bad and just got worse. After his speech, I went outside and threw up in the snow. I was shocked that anyone associated with chiropractic thought it was anything short of a miracle. I was stunned that anyone would try to teach that chiropractic was limited in any way. I made up my mind that day that I was leaving New York Chiropractic College, and going back to Georgia.

I was pretty confident about my decision, but I still had to go home and break it to my wife. When I arrived home I laid it out for her. She never said a word, she just looked at me and smiled. We would've left that day, but the college wouldn't refund my money. I'd also missed the beginning of the first quarter of chiropractic college in Georgia, so I decided to stay for the semester.

It was a real eye opener. It was a new and terrible way to look at our beautiful art of chiropractic. Even now, I can't find words for the abomination that they were teaching. One year to the day I found myself exactly where I started - in Georgia, a place I swore I'd never go again. I even tried to move back to the dilapidated Barclay Arms Apartments, but after one look my wife said absolutely not!

In several ways, my one year in exile was a blessing in disguise. When other students complained about parking or other issues at school, I knew how unimportant these minor issues really were. I would spend the next fourteen quarters at chiropractic college feeling blessed to be there every day.

During the first few weeks at college we all got to know one another, but I hadn't met Liam yet. One of our first classes was CPR. At our college, grades were posted on what was called the "Wailing Wall." You looked up your number and got to see your grade. Then, depending on what it was, you either jumped for joy or cried out in misery. Our first exam in CPR was a twenty question true or false. When our scores were posted, I ran down to the wall and elbowed my way up – I scored a fifteen out of twenty. I was elated! I passed the first exam! I took it as a sign that I would make it at chiropractic college.

When I came back down to earth, I noticed a tall slim guy make his way up to the wall. I saw him slide his finger along the Plexiglas cover, and then I saw his face. At first he looked crushed, then angry. He quickly turned his back, then turned around and looked at the board again.

"I knew it! I just knew it." he said.

"What is the matter with you?" I asked.

"I got one wrong! I knew the right answer, but then I changed it!"

I laughed.

"We have a long way to go until graduation. If you don't relax, never mind straight A's, you might die of an ulcer."

Now he laughed, and introduced himself, and a long lasting friendship was born.

The desire for perfection has driven Liam all the years I've known him. The intense desire to master the situation at all costs has produced the greatest chiropractor of our generation. Starting at chiropractic college was like entering a new world. The other students were the most loving, caring people I'd ever met. The feeling was so infectious that you couldn't help but be in love with chiropractic.

College was set up in such a way that you immediately became immersed in the hands-on of chiropractic. We were given a deep vision and appreciation of our history and philosophy. We were shown the deep commitment to the value of life. We were taught the core values that stand in any profession. We were given the realization that we are here to help others.

The college motto was "give for the sake of giving, love for the sake of loving, and serve for the sake of serving." Dr. B.J. Palmer taught "Get the big idea and all else follows." The college's founder, Dr. Sid Williams, taught "Get the big idea and be of service." Chiropractic was a science, art, and philosophy that if applied correctly could change humanity.

We were taught that just a single chiropractic adjustment can help another human being live a happy, productive life. Chiropractic brings light to the darkness, helping a person live normally again. We were taught that adjusting the vertebral subluxation was the single most important thing we could do for our mother, father, son, daughter, friends, neighbors and clients alike.

We were further taught about the insidious effects of a drug abused society. We were warned in advance, and have since seen the drug companies' true goal. Driven by greed and corporate profits, they are gradually getting every man, woman and child on drugs for a lifetime, from cradle to grave.

It starts with vaccinations at birth, behavior modification pills during adolescence, followed by blood pressure and cholesterol pills, and more behavior-modifying drugs during our middle years. For its final act, Big Pharma really pours it on in our golden years. A barrage of drugs, shots and surgeries are force fed on society, with massive media and government sponsored health (sales) campaigns. Some may read this and call us cultist and reactionary, but we are in a true war for humanity. Imagine, humanity undrugged, and living life to its full potential!

Chiropractic is playing a huge role in this evolution and transformation of health care. Usually when I discuss chiropractic care for a lifetime with people I am met with confusion, disbelief or outright hostility. It never ceases to amaze me that people will ingest and inject drugs from cradle to grave, but resist a spinal adjustment. Chiropractic is the single most important health discovery since 1895.

Our school had an excellent system of technique clubs for its students to learn the art of chiropractic efficiently, in a stress-free, loving environment. These clubs were an integral part of the college experience. You could learn as much as you wanted about individual chiropractic techniques. Clubs were sanctioned by the college, and run by senior students with a faculty member at the head. There are so many great techniques that it would take a lifetime to master them all. Students had the ability to learn, try, and experiment with the ideas, values, and physical requirements of many different techniques.

I was blessed because I became interested in upper cervical technique in first quarter. I had great results for myself with full spine and upper cervical, so there was never any doubt in my mind that all the techniques worked. I was fortunate to be in a place where I could be immersed in so many different techniques during fourteen quarters of study.

One of the important extras we received at college was assembly. Dr. Sid would have the whole school assemble so he could explain chiropractic to us. His message of service was as important as our classroom education.

It was during my first quarter that I met Dr. Sid outside of class. I've always felt privileged to have been a student while Dr. Sid was the leading force at the college. I was also extremely lucky to have many personal conversations with him while I was a student.

My first meeting with Dr. Sid was the most memorable one. One of the remnants I had from the days of my scrap metal business was my large German Shepard named Shadow. Shadow guarded the trucks when we had jobs in tough neighborhoods, and she watched over me and others when we went into supposedly abandoned buildings and various other places. She'd mastered the art of dealing with vagrants, squatters and thieves. She'd put on a display of ferocity that got almost anybody to move. In the rare instances that actual physical contact was required, she never hesitated. She protected me many times. In the course of keeping me safe, she bit many people, and sustained a few injuries herself. She was fully capable of taking care of herself, and us, in almost any situation.

When I started at chiropractic college, there was a lot of internal debate as to whether to take her with me or not. I was doubtful about whether she could adapt to a peaceful existence in urban Atlanta. As usual, Shadow took things into her own paws. As it came closer to the time for me to leave for college, she took to living in my pickup truck. When moving day came, nothing could get her to come out. So by default she became an apartment dog living in Atlanta.

Shadow required a huge amount of physical exercise as well as personal interaction. I often took her to the campus for socialization and some exercise. At that time, the college grounds were still unfinished with many of the fields being mostly mud. During rain storms the river that runs along the lower rugby pitch often overflowed, creating a real mess. It was during one of these major rainstorms that I first personally met Dr. Sid.

Shadow and I were running in a very muddy rugby field. All of a sudden a long white Cadillac pulled up along the field. The window buzzed about a quarter of the way down.

"Hey, are you one of my students?"

I could tell it was Dr. Sid immediately by his voice, and I figured I was in big trouble for making a mud patch out of the rugby pitch. His voice had a slight bite to it and given the circumstances, I could understand why. He seemed clearly annoyed that we were in the field, but before I could even respond, Shadow, hearing the very slight hostility in his voice, launched herself at the opened window of the Cadillac like a guided missile.

She charged the caddy with a full growl, teeth out, hair up, ready to do battle. She put her big wet muddy feet on the window sill of the caddy with her head against the window.

I began to bolt over to the car, "Sorry Dr. Sid, I'll get her!"

Before I could take two steps, the window buzzed all the way down, and out came a hand with a gold ring, fancy watch, starched white shirt and gold cuff links.

"Boy that's a nice dog!" Dr. Sid said, while patting Shadow on the head, giving both of her big ears a big squeeze. Shadow was so surprised she stopped growling and wagged her tail. Shadow stayed up on the door. Dr. Sid reached way out with both hands and gave her a full going over. As I got to the car to give my apologies, Sid cut me off.

"Are you one of my students?"

"Yes sir, Judd Nogrady first quarter!"

He smiled broadly "This is a really nice dog. Good to meet both of you."

With that the window buzzed up and the Caddy glided away.

After many trips to the Wailing Wall, first quarter soon faded, we had a break, and awaited second quarter.

Liam

When I arrived at chiropractic college I had two goals: to become the most proficient student, and to secure work that allowed me to attend chiropractic college while supporting myself financially. I was very fortunate, because soon after I settled into my apartment, I landed a security job at Allied Security, Inc. It was one of the oldest, most respected firms in Atlanta.

Contrary to what I first imagined, the life of an Allied security guard is not all glamour, intrigue, and action. Instead, almost all of my assignments consisted of sitting in an office keeping my eyes on the building after all its inhabitants had gone home. And guess what? Office buildings have a habit of staying just where you put them.

I found the maximum shift guards were allowed to work was twelve hours. I became the twelve hour security shift specialist. I worked twelve hours Saturday, and twelve hours Sunday. "Work" was primarily sitting at a desk, with nobody around me, in almost complete silence. This allowed me to study, study and study.

My objective became to use the twenty-four hours of work every weekend as study time, a time to absolutely master all the material that was presented in class that week. Of course, I studied most nights after class, but the extra twenty-four hours on the weekends gave me the extra edge.

The extra income provided me with much needed financial relief. My parents had helped me with my undergraduate degree, which was a huge financial burden for them. So we decided that any postgraduate work would be my financial responsibility. I knew it was easy to spend someone else's money, while decisions about spending my own would be made with more deliberation. I was determined to keep my loan debt down to an absolute minimum.

My first recollection of Dr. Judd was during a first quarter spinal anatomy class, while taking an exam. For this exam we had to know the origin and insertion of muscles. All this was new to me, and it was very challenging. I'd spent one twelve hour shift memorizing all the muscle names and groups and another shift memorizing every origin, insertion, and action. I had every muscle memorized, and I was ready to ace my first exam.

As I'm sitting at my desk trying to concentrate on the exam, out of the corner of my eye, I saw someone making jerky movements. He started slapping his thigh, then slapping his knee. Next he slapped his knee and followed this by slapping his ankle. It took me a few seconds to figure it out. This maniac was slapping all the origins and insertions and getting the muscle actions. He was so distracting that I was going to raise my hand to ask the instructor to tell him to stop, but then I noticed that this guy was built like a cross between a mountain lion and an orangutan. I decided to re-focus on my own exam.

I made a mental note never to sit near him during an exam again. I made another mental note to avoid him all together because he was obviously an over-muscled nut job. I was soon to learn that first impressions can be wrong. Our friendship would get us both through school and launch us into a beautiful life of abundance through service to humanity, with the power and principles of chiropractic.

It's funny when you think about it. I'd made a mental note to avoid Dr. Judd, but after the next exam he approached me. I'd just seen my results from a CPR exam and I was upset, stressed, and disappointed with my score. I wanted to be the best chiropractor that had ever walked the face of the planet. I'd mistakenly adopted the belief system that those who excelled in academics were those that were going to be the greatest chiropractors in the world. This false belief was behind my ridiculous antics at missing one question on this exam.

All this frustration came pouring out at exactly the moment Dr. Judd saw me. He decided I needed a reality check. I'll never forget the way he asked what was the matter with me. It really wasn't a question, but rather a declaration that he knew I was over reacting. My first response was to tell him to mind his business. However, after his antics in spinal anatomy class, I was rather intimidated by him, which is a nice way of saying scared.

I answered that I'd missed one question on the exam, and was angry because I'd answered correctly but then changed the answer at the last minute. He smiled. That smile taught me that while my habit of trying to study for perfection does guarantee good grades, it's just as important not to take yourself too damn seriously.

Soon after this initial meeting, Judd proposed that we set up a study team. There were many students doing group studies. They usually start out with some studying and then develop into pizza and beer parties. We wanted nothing to do with that. If we ever played hooky or took time away from studying, it was to escape to the north Georgia Mountains or to roam the canyons in Alabama. (Nothing is better than good friends taking hiking trips, which are great fun, and just as important, inexpensive).

It was during our team study sessions that I realized Judd and I were becoming the study "Dream Team'. I was a good student by nature and had a lifetime of good study habits. Judd, on the other hand, was a collection of opposites. He was the most committed student I'd ever met, but possibly one of the worst test takers. He certainly knew the material, but a multiple choice question could outfox him more often than not.

Due to having dyslexia, he had a difficult time writing notes during lectures. So instead of writing, he would just sit and listen. He retained an extraordinary amount of material. On top of this, he'd tape every lecture and write out every word the teacher said. Together, we'd decode the teacher's message.

On many occasions, we'd spend countless hours studying certain aspects of a particular course, and then the teacher would focus the exam on another part, leaving us looking foolish and unprepared. During these frustrating study times Judd and I began to double our efforts. We decided to let nothing stand in our way of academic excellence.

As time went on, we began to gain the reputation as being the academically gifted ones in class. I'd receive phone calls from members of my class, asking me to explain a difficult concept that an instructor had outlined, or to provide answers to tricky homework problems. I'd go over with them why an answer was the right answer.

One really had to know the concepts behind the questions in order to choose the right answer.

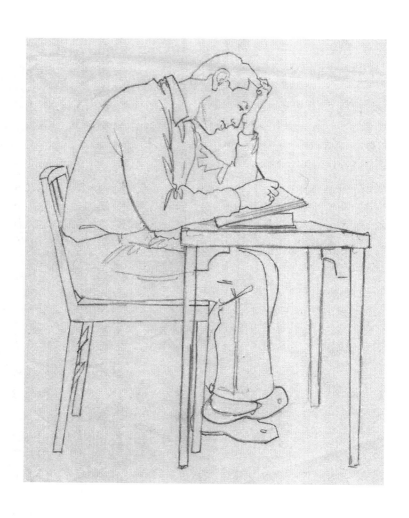

CHAPTER 6

How many more subjects?

Judd

The courses at chiropractic college are more demanding than most people realize. They required a level of study I hadn't mastered yet. My current M.O. was to tape the class and listen with unbroken concentration because I didn't have to bother writing notes. After class or in the evening I'd replay the lecture and write it out word for word. A fifty minute lecture took about two hours; similarly a two hour lecture took about four hours.

While I'm sure I didn't get the best grades of all the students at my college, I'm certain I had the best notes, and I'm absolutely sure no one knew the material better than I did. I believe my method of studying resulted in excellent long term retention. Even today, I remember long passages of notes that I wrote out years ago.

By sheer happenstance, Liam's Wailing Wall number was directly above mine, a fact I learned on that first CPR exam. I couldn't help but notice that he always scored in the extremely high 90's. Unfortunately, my grades were never nearly as high. I knew I had to make some kind of change. I loved chiropractic, but I was barely passing. Without a degree, I was near useless in the world of chiropractic. Putting more time in would have been impossible. I had to learn a better way. I decided to seek out Liam for some extra help.

I was never a person to be indirect, so after class I laid it all out for him. I would supply the best notes he'd ever seen if he would show me how to study more effectively. To seal the deal, I brought my notes from the last lecture, all eighteen pages, handwritten, single spaced, written verbatim, every single word out of the professors mouth. Liam took one look and agreed.

He certainly didn't need my notes, but I'd like to think he knew a good deal when he saw one. My notes must've made lectures more enjoyable for him. Whatever the reason, I'm glad he agreed, because he was an excellent study partner.

When the third quarter started there was a palpable tension in the air and around our class. In the beginning of third quarter, we were informed that we were required to take the first part of National Board exams next quarter. From now on, in addition to our regular heavy course load, we'd be studying for "boards." It's here that I can say that our full attention to becoming the world's greatest chiropractors started to become a secondary priority. Instead, we were redirected to becoming masters of passing the boards.

It's easy to think that passing boards is just one hoop to jump through to become a chiropractor, but I always resented it a waste of time. It would've been great to use the time, energy, and money spent on boards to learn information that could've actually been a benefit to our practice members. I think the best way to fully explain this is to give an actual example of a board question. This was question number 46 on a National Board exam for chiropractic:

In a sewage plant an effluent lagoon is used for

    a. settling sewage waste

    b. drinking water

    c. solid waste only

    d. liquid waste only

I think this question puts to rest the relevance and the importance the National Board people put on chiropractic. (In case you are wondering, the correct answer is "a.") I could and may write a separate book on the National Board system, but at this point let's get on with becoming a chiropractor. On a separate note, this question did get a laugh from some of the guys that work in the sewage department in my town. They say everyone calls the effluent lagoon the "shit pit."

Liam

One of the best ideas at school was the opportunity to be paired with a student chiropractor. All students received free adjustments. During my time at college I was fortunate to have been paired with two dedicated, yet very different student chiropractors. My first student doctor was Obi Chinakwe from Nigeria. He was a sharp dresser with a great mind, and a contagious smile. He was meticulous with his adjustment technique. After my first adjustment with him I had a smile from ear to ear. I walked across campus to my first class with a great feeling knowing that my body was functioning at its best! It was unbelievable to me that the school provided chiropractic care for free to all students.

Getting chiropractic care throughout college helped me handle the stressful days that college can dish out. Without it, I never would've endured the hectic pace of school. To this day, regular care helps me live my life at hyper-drive.

My next student chiropractor was Todd Harkleroad from Kentucky, a dedicated Gonstead Chiropractor. He had an unbelievable understanding of spinal mechanics, was a brilliant adjuster, and his proficiency set the bar high for all students. Todd was a real character. He was a heavy smoker and always smelled like cigarette smoke. I didn't understand half of what he said because of his thick accent but his sense of humor, and his absolute dedication to giving the best adjustment possible, made him a great student chiropractor.

In my travels, I've learned that in certain parts of the southern United States, many people thought nothing of their doctors smoking. Being from New Jersey, however, I found it shocking.

These two student chiropractors from completely different parts of the world inspired me to be my best. It was great to be part of a profession that had plenty of room for different personalities. It was also exciting to be part of a worldwide group all united in one cause.

I once heard Dr. Bill Decken, a world renowned chiropractic philosophy professor at Sherman College of Chiropractic, describe chiropractic schooling as schizophrenic in nature. We enter chiropractic college to learn chiropractic and are quickly given a medical education. What amazed me about chiropractic school is how much focus there is on learning medicine. When I was in school, I thought that because the accrediting scheme required these courses, then they must somehow be vital to the practice of chiropractic. I was absolutely stunned when I learned that nothing can be further from the truth. Roughly seventy-five percent of what is taught in "accredited" chiropractic schools is almost completely irrelevant to the modern practice of chiropractic. This watering down and diluting of the true chiropractic message is a huge disservice to chiropractors and the people they care for.

Can you imagine going to your dentist to have a prostate exam? How about a vaginal check-up? How about a blood pressure check, urinalysis, heart exam and a resulting medical diagnosis? Chiropractors in current Council on Chiropractic Education (CCE) accredited schools are trained to do these things every day. I've been going to the dentist regularly for over thirty years, but the dentist has always checked my teeth and my teeth only. The dentist seems to know that good dental care is vital to good health, no matter what the rest of your body is doing. Their focus has not changed. Maybe this is why they continue to grow and flourish. We need to be focused on the message that the body always functions better without nerve interference, period!

I resigned myself to the fact that much of my education was sadly going to be in things not pertaining to the practice of chiropractic. Our school was wonderful because although they taught these CCE required courses, the school's leaders always took us aside and showed us the real power of chiropractic. We had a president, professors, and fellow students who had a wealth of experience serving the masses. They made us keenly aware of our awesome responsibility, to chiropractic and to the people. They removed our blinders to the medical system and let us see what Big Pharma truly stood for. They, like us, had their hands bound. They were playing the CCE game of hide the truth.

The more I learned about the true power of chiropractic, the more school became a game. In order to gain the privilege to liberate lives through the power of chiropractic, I was going to have to master the CCE game of hide the chiropractic. Judd and I always took the approach that we'd learn whatever the CCE wanted no matter how irrelevant in nature. We were determined to master the information through disciplined study. We knew this was an unfortunate obstacle that we had to overcome to receive our diplomas and live the chiropractic dream.

Judd and I made another steadfast vow: if either one of us should ever deviate from the path, the other would give a frightful beating. This was scarier for me than him! We also made a promise that we'd do whatever it took to become successful chiropractors, so that one day we could come back and help change the chiropractic educational system that was full of moral decay and corruption. As I write this book, my heart is glad that we have started down this path.

As we progressed in our education, we became eligible to begin taking our chiropractic National Boards. There are now four parts to the National Boards. Each one is a testament to how far from reality the CCE has become when left to its own devices. One of the goals of this book is to cause chiropractors to wake up and realize that our profession has been high-jacked. My hope is that the government or perhaps a media organization appoints someone to investigate the validity and relevance of the information that is tested by the National Board of Chiropractic Examiners. Bringing light to this process would cause much needed reform in a system that is incongruent with the practice of modern chiropractic.

What makes boards difficult for many is the simple fact that the information tested many times has nothing to do with the practice of chiropractic.

Liam

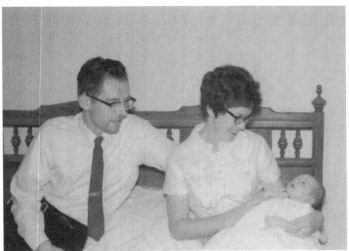

1969 – Coming home to Freehold, New Jersey, USA with Mom and Dad.

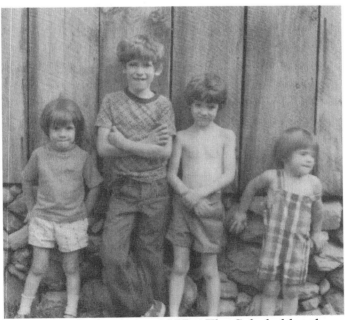

1977 – The Schubel brothers
Middletown Springs, Vermont, USA.

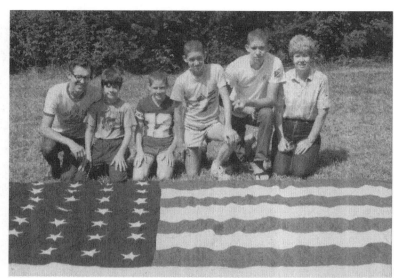

1983 – Ear accentuating hair cuts and family patriotism at the Schubel summer home in Middletown Springs, Vermont, USA.

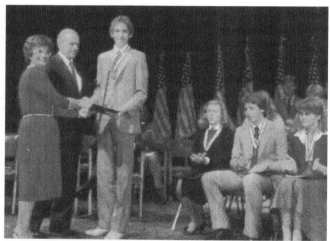

1986 – Receiving the Bronze Congressional Award from New Jersey Congressman Hon. James J. Howard.

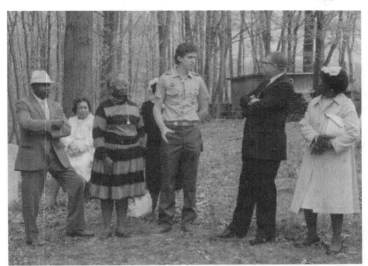

1987 – Eagle Scout project, restoring African American
Civil War Veteran's Cemetary in Freehold, New Jersey.

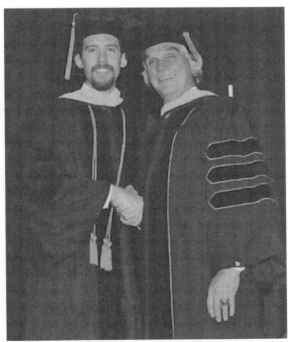

1995 – Chiropractic School Graduation with
Founder and President of Life College
Dr. Sid E. Williams.

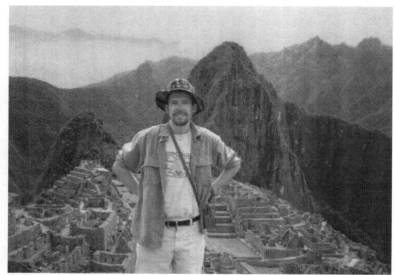

1997 – Macchu Piccu, Peru

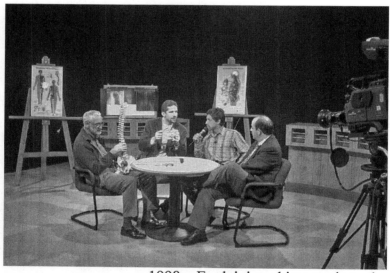

1998 – Explaining chiropractic to the
people of Peru on live television.

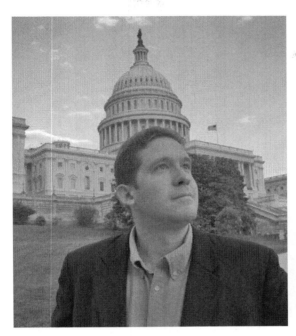

2000 –
Participating
in the political
process –
Washington
D.C., USA.

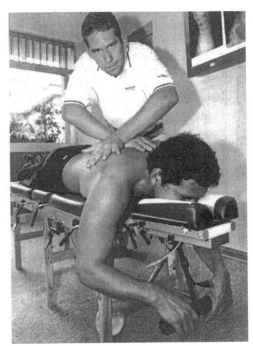

2001 – Adjusting
1,000 practice
members a week in
my prime in Peru.

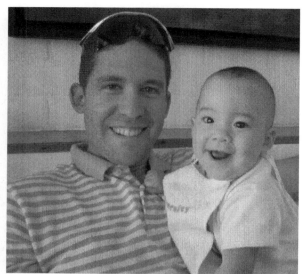

2002 – My daughter Maryanne and I
at Pulpos Beach House, Peru

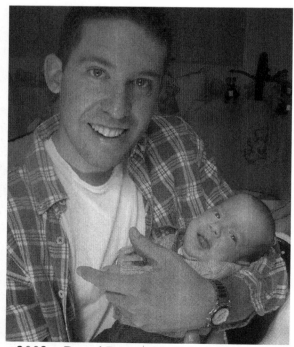

2002 – Proud Papa with Schubelnator Jr. –
Pulpos Beach House, Peru

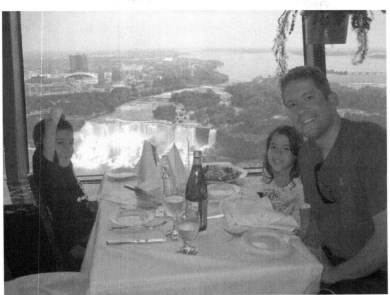

2009 – Niagra Falls, Canada with Liam Jr. and Maryanne.

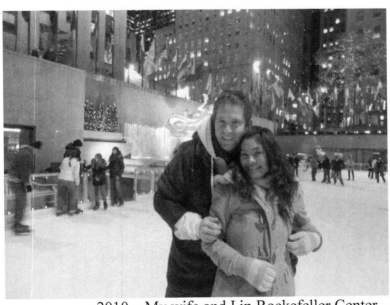

2010 – My wife and I in Rockefeller Center –
New York City, USA.

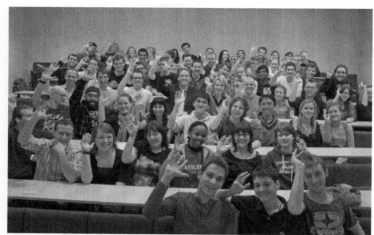

2010 – Schubelnator World Chiropractic College Tour –
Wales, United Kingdom.

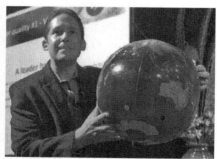

2010 – Speaking at New
Zealand Chiropractic College

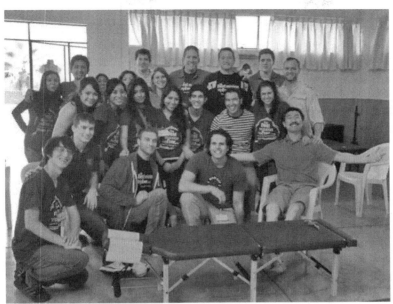

2010 – The Best Mission Trip Ever!
Team of Servants from around the world, Lima, Peru

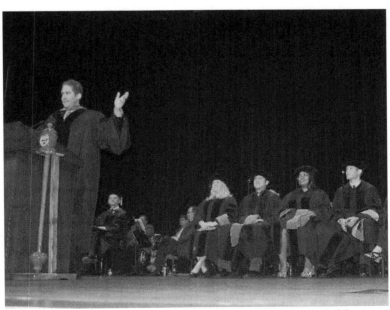

2011 – Commencement Address at
Sherman College of Chiropractic

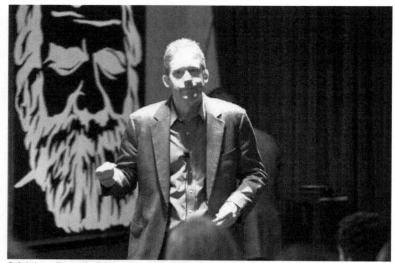

2011 – Dead Chiropractic Society Clubhouse California, USA.

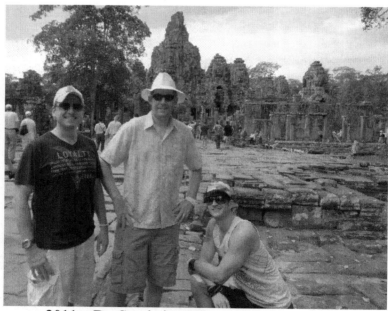

2011 – Dr. Sontheimer, Dr. Schubel and Dr. Taylor – World Chiropractic Tri-force, Angor Wat, Cambodia.

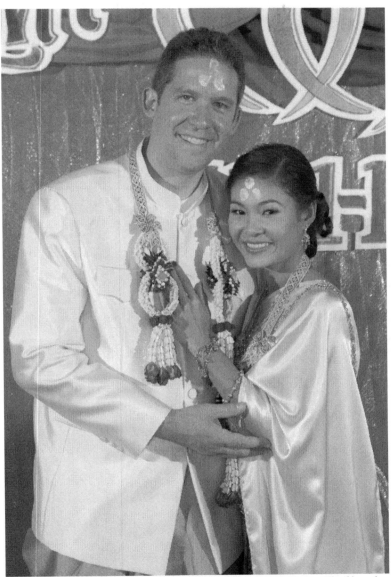

2011 – The King and The Ning, Aranyaprathet, Thailand.

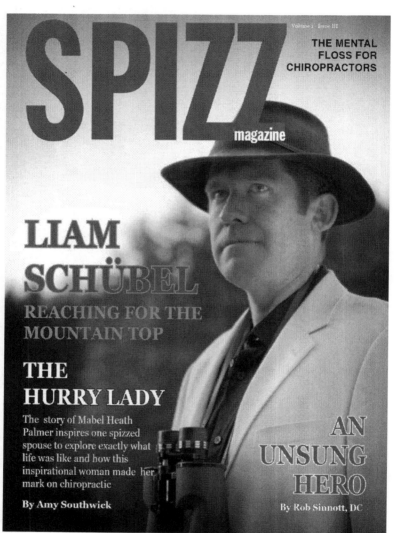

SPIZZ magazine

Volume I · Issue III

THE MENTAL FLOSS FOR CHIROPRACTORS

LIAM SCHÜBEL

REACHING FOR THE MOUNTAIN TOP

THE HURRY LADY

The story of Mabel Heath Palmer inspires one spizzed spouse to explore exactly what life was like and how this inspirational woman made her mark on chiropractic

By Amy Southwick

AN UNSUNG HERO

By Rob Sinnott, DC

2012 – Front cover of world renowned chiropractic periodicals – Spizz Magazine.

Judd

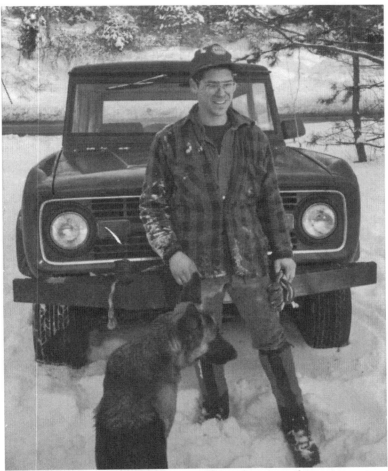

One of my early jobs was off road tow and recovery.

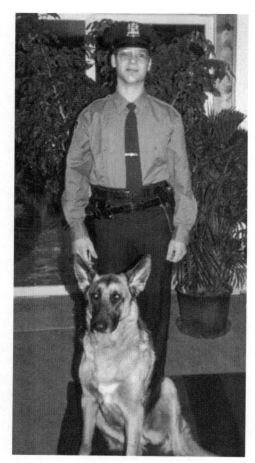

Here I am One of
New York City's
Finest.

The crew from the
days of hauling
scrap metal.
"When you're
little it pays to
have big friends."

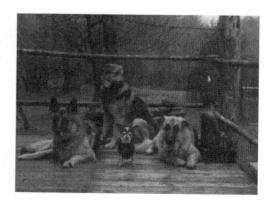

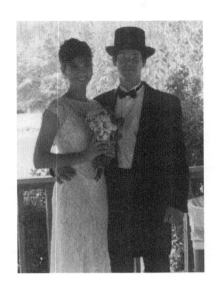

One of the best days
of my life.

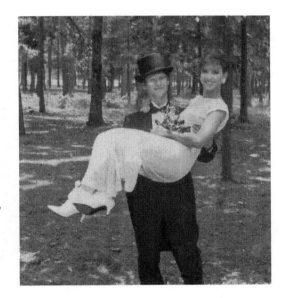

Happy I am married,
and happy I'm
healthy enough to
carry my beautiful
bride!

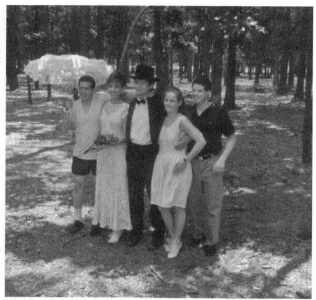

(Left to right) My brother Dr. Alec Nogrady, my wife
Dr. Veronica Nogrady, me, my sister Dr. Jill Nogrady,
And my brother Dr. Adam Nogrady.

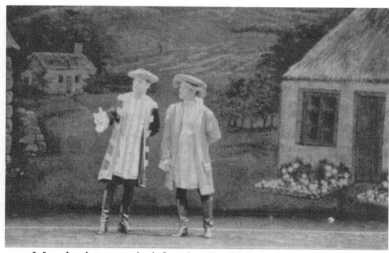

Me playing a nobel for the Georgia ballet. It's amazing
what a college student will do to make money.
$50 a night was big money!

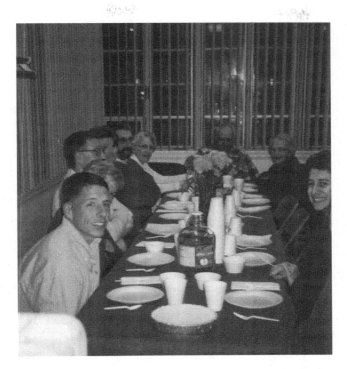

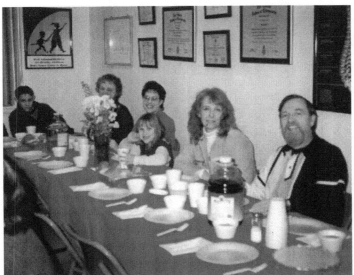

During the first few years I was in practice we always had practice members come to the office for a traditional Thanksgiving dinner. This year we served over 300.

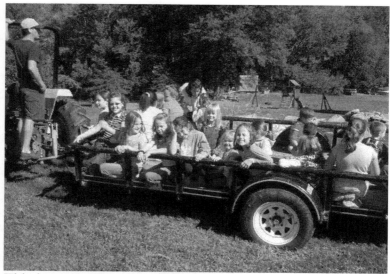

This is our hayless hay ride for the kids – hayless because so many of them are in the process of overcoming asthma and a variety of other issues.

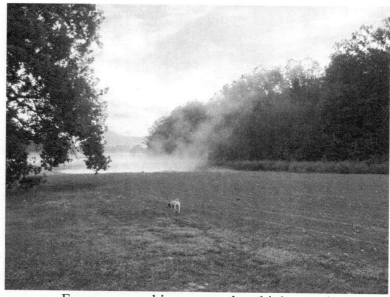

For any new chiropractor that thinks starting a new practice is challenging – try farming. This is going to be five acres of radishes.

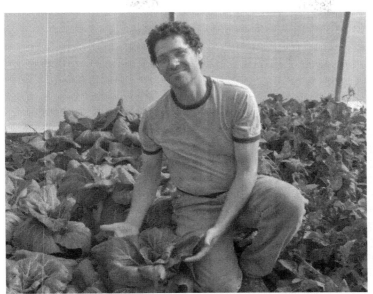

It's great when crops actually grow. Here's a nice
bunch of Bok-Choi.

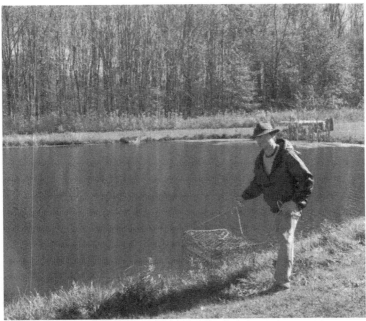

Getting back to the land just happens –
here I'm setting fish traps on the farm.

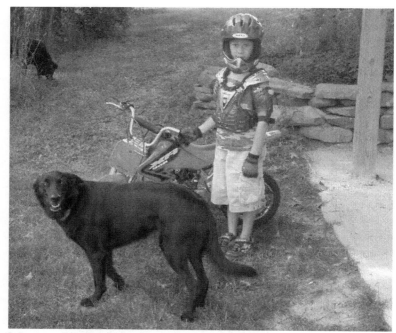

My son Jacob with our pal Lola on his 6th birthday, trying out his present from dad.

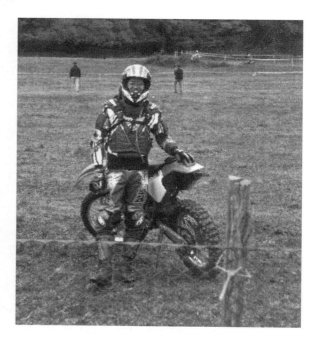

Motorcycle racing is absolutely great – but I don't recommend it for any chiropractor.

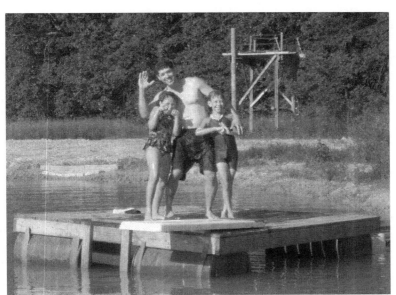

At the pond with my daughter Montana and son Jake.
They thought swimming here was the best until
they saw their first snapping turtle.

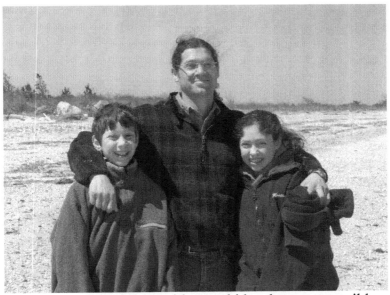

Spend time with your kids whenever possible –
they grow up so fast!

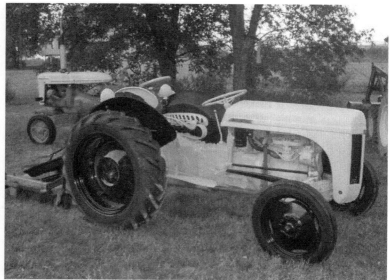

I've always loved restoring old machinery. These tractors are hard-working antiques - a 1948 Farmall and a 1950 TO 20 Ferguson.

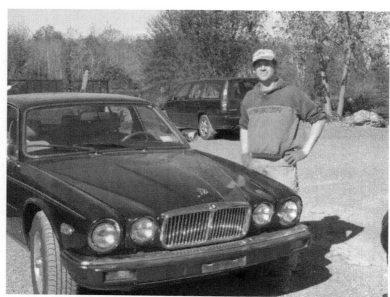

My wife always thought I was crazy for restoring old machines until I gave here this beautifully restored Jaguar for our 19th wedding anniversary.

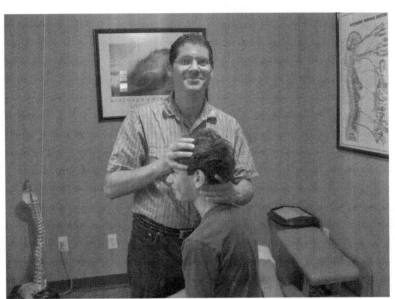

Taking care of infants and children is the backbone of my practice. Here is my son showing a timid new patient how it is done.

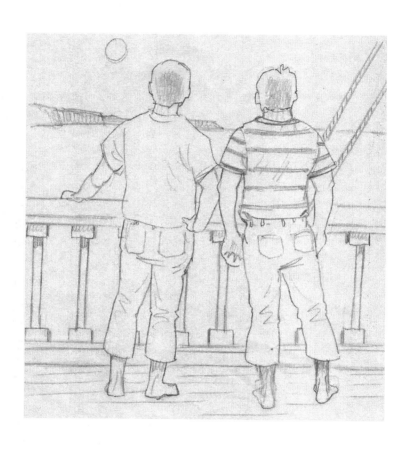

CHAPTER 7

We get to see the people

Judd

Liam and I spent six weeks reviewing for boards, after which we signed up for "Irene." Irene is a separate company that has been copied but never duplicated, that preps chiropractors for the national boards. They and others have classes for every part of the boards. They have it so completely dialed in that many offer money back guarantees if you fail.

I feel almost any person with average intelligence could pass any board exam, without ever setting so much as a big toe into any chiropractic classroom or college, after spending two weeks with Irene and her notes! I'm happy to report that I must have at least average intelligence, because I passed the exams, and it should go without saying that Liam passed also.

Part one of the board exam was a huge load on my shoulders. With the exam finished I breathed a sigh of relief. At that time, I thought if you failed you were thrown out of school. I've subsequently learned that the only consequence to failing board exams is that you have to pay an exorbitant fee to the national board cartel, but you can retake the exam again and again, as many times as necessary. This is why ninety-nine percent of all students eventually pass them.

As part of the license requirement for New York State, one needs to take a PT (physical therapy) course and a board sponsored PT exam. At that time, our college didn't allow PT on campus because it is unrelated to chiropractic. We paid National College to come down and give us an abridged version of their PT class which allowed us to take the PT board exam.

This whole system is a sham. Instead of taking three years of PT at National College, which is famous for their physical therapy modalities, it can be done in two weeks in a cramped auditorium. The end result is that I have a degree from National College in PT, and my degree has been verified by the national boards. However, I've NEVER actually touched any of the various machines used in PT, never administered PT, never seen PT done, yet I am considered trained by the best college for PT, and I'm certified by the national boards to do PT!

After having jumped through the hoops of national boards, the next big step is clinic. I couldn't imagine a more exciting and rewarding time in life. It was great to start helping people with chiropractic.

One of the rewarding things about our college clinic experience was that it was "trial by fire." In the clinic, it was just you, the patient, and an adjusting table. One quickly learned how important good adjusting skills are, and the value of a good chiropractic analysis. Being a competent adjuster was second to being a competent palpator. Knowing where the subluxation is, and that you've corrected it, has to be the best feeling on earth! The how, why, where, and when to adjust is what colleges need to focus on most.

Starting clinic is a real eye opener. I assumed the population in general would just somehow know what a good guy I was and flock to me as a chiropractic healer. I'd accepted chiropractic in full faith. I'd embraced the "big idea" so much so, that I imagined I'd be so busy that I'd have to be open seven days a week to take care of people.

Unfortunately, back on earth, my prospective clients were generally not as enthusiastic as I was. I figured it was the clinic environment, or the fact that I was still just a student doctor. Nothing is sadder than an eager chiropractor with no people to adjust. I was stunned. The idea of having to get people to come for adjustments had never occurred to me. The idea that you would have to explain chiropractic over and over was such a shock that I briefly considered quitting. Chiropractic was so beautiful that the idea of having to sell it was horrible.

Liam stepped in and helped to lift my spirits. His feeling was that people just don't know about chiropractic yet. His opinion was that it was our job to inform the public as many times as possible about the tremendous life changing benefits of chiropractic care, and to open their eyes to the danger of using drugs for every symptom. Dr. Liam took his spine and gave mini lay lectures everywhere he went. As a result of getting out and spreading the word, he attracted so many people to the clinic that he sailed through, and helped me achieve my clinic requirements as well.

Although clinic was an incredibly fun and exciting experience, I really yearned to get out into the real world and open my office. I envisioned at least 100 chairs in my waiting room. With clinic requirements finished, there were still a few hurdles remaining. Exit exams were some of the most intriguing and challenging exams I've ever taken.

All exams were videotaped, and you were put into real life situations with another student playing the part of the practice member. After the exam, you had the opportunity to watch your performance, or lack thereof. It was a real eye opener. Points were scored based on bedside manner, thoroughness, and chiropractic analysis. Lastly, you had to explain in detail how, when, and why you were going to adjust, and what adjusting technique you were going to use. The exams were tough but fair, and they exactly mirrored real life situations.

I'm happy to say I passed all my exams and was ready to graduate! I had six months of police academy training, three years of pre-chiropractic college, one semester at New York Chiropractic College, and fourteen quarters at chiropractic college in Georgia (roughly four years). I passed three National Board exams, adjusted 350 people at the clinic, and passed all clinic entrance exams, all clinic exit exams, and final exams.

Yet, there was still more testing before I could bring chiropractic to the world. I had to take the New York State exam. At that time, every state had their own exam which was required in order to get a license. The New York State Chiropractic Licensing exam was given at the New York Chiropractic College. It was a strange feeling to be finishing exactly where I started.

Happily, the New York exam was very much like the school clinic exam. It was straightforward, with direct doctor practice member contact. All questions were asked by an instructor. During the exam, the chiropractic practice member was a prospective chiropractor just like me. When I was done being tested, I became a practice member for them.

By chance, I was paired with a recent graduate of New York Chiropractic College. She was the doctor first and I was the mock patient. I played a mother bringing in a six year old with asthma. When she entered the room, she looked every part the professional. She was poised, polished, and very doctoral looking. She asked how I was and what she could help with today.

As I read off the conditions on the card, and the age of my child, you could see the blood drain from her face. The examiner, an older chiropractor, seemed like a nice guy. He sensed her anxiety, so he asked her very gently, did she need me to re-read the card or explain further? She looked around the room like she wanted to bolt. Her answer so surprised the both of us that the examiner looked at me for an explanation!

On the verge of tears, she blurted out that she would not adjust a child, and she would then explain to the mother that chiropractic was not used in asthma cases. Further, she went on to say she would report her for child abuse if she didn't seek proper medical care. This poor girl then tried to compose herself by adding that if the mother desired, she could give the child a physical exam, but only if the mother would sign a consent form first.

The examiner looked completely stunned. He looked around the room, then at me. I stood there with my mouth opened. He asked her, why would you ask a practice member to sign a consent form if she was bringing the child in for chiropractic care? Obviously she wanted the chiropractor to examine the child. Well, this put her over the edge. The tears rolled down her cheeks. She responded, "why would anyone bring a child to the chiropractor?!"

The sad part is that this girl was not a bad person, she'd just never been taught how to be a chiropractor. I felt bad for her, but had to stay focused on passing my own exam. She was given a few moments to compose herself, as she still had to play practice member for me. She got my card, and as she began reading it, she seemed flabbergasted. Her card said she was bringing in her five month old with problems nursing.

The instructor asked were there any exams I'd perform first before my chiropractic exam. I was never so happy in my life with my education. I quickly explained how I would palpate an infant. I demonstrated the proper procedure for subluxation detection on an infant as defined by the protocol of the adjusting technique I was going to use. The examiner gave me a big smile. Proceed "doctor." At that moment I knew I had done it. I explained my chiropractic findings. I explained that I would fingertip toggle with a child's toggle board. This was all done verbatim as taught at our school. Needless to say, I passed my final hurdle. Liam and I had a great time at graduation.

After graduation we chose separate paths. Dr. Liam went off to South America to practice, and I went to exotic upstate New York. Even though we were separated by 7,000 miles, we were entwined by a deep desire to provide chiropractic service and a love for our fellow humans.

Liam

With all the studying, boards, and bookwork, the chance to work with people couldn't come fast enough for me. I was dying for some hands on experience!

Not everyone in chiropractic education and legislation has lost their minds. I had quite a positive experience as a student visiting the state of Alabama. Some states allow you to take your chiropractic licensure exam while you're a student, and Alabama was one of them. A whole bunch of us drove over to Birmingham, Alabama in a convoy accompanied by a few of our southern colleagues to vouch for us. We checked into our hotel, and that evening we were surprisingly invited to a cocktail hour to meet the Alabama Chiropractic State Board of Examiners.

The leader of the group introduced himself and the other members of the board, and told us that he was excited for us, and that Alabama needed more good chiropractors. He wished us luck on the exam, and after a while we all retired to our rooms early. I was very impressed with their southern hospitality.

The next day the testing began. I had some real characters testing me. One of the examiners was actually smoking a cigarette while administering the test! The exam was very straightforward, and for the most part was a chiropractic exam with relevant spinal X-rays, adjusting, and patient care scenarios.

Almost everyone passed the test because we had been trained to be chiropractors, and chiropractic is what the test was based on. I later learned that Alabama was a chiropractic friendly board. Believe it or not, there are many state chiropractic boards that are unfriendly towards chiropractors. Notorious states at that time were Florida (people joked it was the Florida Medical exam not the Florida Chiropractic exam), California, and New Jersey. The exams in these states were very difficult because again the material that they tested was mainly medical.

These states made their exams very difficult to pass under the auspices of protecting the public, but what's become clear is the following: in states where there are a lot of chiropractors, perceived competition is fierce. These states often times use extremely difficult exams, and stifling regulations and paperwork requirements in order to make it difficult for new chiropractors to enter that state. What's always saddened me is how they justify this obvious territorial protectionism.

I have fond memories of being a student chiropractor at college. They were probably some of the best moments in my life. It was great to finally be able to help others. Finally, I was allowed to apply some of the things we were learning in the classroom in order to improve the quality of life for my fellow human beings. We were given blue clinic jackets to indicate that we were ready to work in the college clinic, and I must tell you that from that point on, I began to feel like I really was a chiropractor. I was so proud of how far I'd come, and how many obstacles I'd overcome in order to gain the privilege of helping others with chiropractic.

When I was in school, our college had a requirement that we had to adjust 350 people in order to gain experience and demonstrate basic proficiency before we could graduate. In addition to the 350 practice member adjustments, we also had to do a certain amount of urinalysis and two hour physical exams! To this day I don't fully understand what the relevance of all this was to the modern practice of chiropractic.

During the two hour exam we checked most every organ system including the heart, and looked at the shape of their retinas! Who the heck came up with this idea? I can imagine the cardiologist eaves dropping in on a chiropractic heart exam and then imagine his horror as we pronounce the heart "fit" when he, a cardiologist, takes twice the time and twice the investigation, not to mention a stress test and blood work before he offers any opinion.

But alas, we listen with our quivering stethoscope and pronounce heart wellness.

We were also required to do eye exams. Our eye exams were done without the aid of the drug Atropine which allows the eye to dilate. One check with any qualified eye doctor will set you straight to the fact that there can be absolutely no quality exam without this drug. It makes no sense why the accrediting agencies want chiropractic students to check eyes. I thought we were experts in the spine and nervous system!!

Needless to say, because of all the unnecessary paperwork and irrelevant tests many students quickly became despondent. I believe many students have their chiropractic flame extinguished by going through this process! In spite of all this negativity, I was going to try to be the most successful chiropractic student I could be. The founder and president of our college taught us that with our hands, hearts, minds and voice we could help the whole world to function and heal optimally. I took him very seriously (and still do). This knowledge propelled me to be the most successful student chiropractor in my class.

Many students had a tough time meeting their clinic requirements for many reasons. The most popular reasons were fear and negativity. They spent their days complaining about the system we had to practice in, or complaining about the community's reluctance to come in and see a beginning chiropractor. Many were too shy to open up and share the chiropractic story or to educate the people about how chiropractic could greatly benefit their lives.

I must admit that internally, I had many of the same thoughts that they did. I've always been uncomfortable with sales or selling things, and the thought of trying to sell people on the idea to come to see me, the newbie in the college clinic, made me painfully uncomfortable. I knew from experience, however, that whatever you fear the most in the world is exactly what you need to do if you want to advance in life. To grow, you must face the fear if you want to get past it.

One of my book mentors, Eleanor Roosevelt, used to say, "That which we fear and confront is what makes us stronger." I knew innately that this was what was going to make me stronger as a communicator, as a chiropractor, and as a human being. Love for chiropractic and my fellow humans would be the fuel that would propel me to lose the fear of confronting people. The experience of overcoming these fears turned out to be one of the biggest factors to the success I'd experience later on in my career as a chiropractor.

I didn't know anybody in Georgia outside of the students at school. I'm not the kind of guy that makes friends easily and am not very socially active, either. The question I asked myself back then was, how am I going to find people to come into the clinic to get adjusted by Liam Schübel, the inexperienced chiropractic student?

The first thing I needed to do was to get my thoughts and ideas organized. As I've learned over the years, everything that you manifest in your life is a direct result of your thoughts and actions. If I was going to achieve excellence rather than struggle as many others did, I was going to have to think and act differently. The first thing that I decided to do was to list all the reasons why a person would want to come to see me in the clinic:

1. They had vertebral subluxations that were limiting their capacity to heal and function optimally.

2. There was no one else who would care for them like I would.
3. Because we were students, the office fee was one third of a regular chiropractic fee.
4. They'd get the most thorough medical exam in their life performed by a chiropractic student.

I made sure I turned every negative into a positive.

From this point on, I decided to look at the clinic with new eyes and thoughts. Thinking in this fashion took me from a position of begging people to come in, and moved me to a position of offering a valuable service at an extremely reasonable price. I managed to completely convince myself that if people didn't take advantage of my offer, then they were missing out, not me.

Now that I had the mindset down, I needed to draw up a plan of action. I was assigned to the north clinic which was in a more rural area then the main clinic. I found a Georgia map and then figured out where the people who lived and worked in this area would be. I drew a red circle of twenty miles in radius around the north clinic and decided that this was going to be my neighborhood.

Many chiropractors in the profession limit their vision to people in pain. Let's lay aside the moral issue of how wrong it is to ignore the asymptomatic population that has subluxations, like infants and young children. Most chiropractors agree that vertebral subluxations are silent killers because of the damage they do to the nervous system without causing any pain. Why then don't we inform the public en masse like dentists have done with cavity prevention?

When people begin to suffer from back or neck pain, their first choice to treat it is most often medicine. Taking pills is by far the cheapest way to treat back and neck pain in the short term. Of course, taking pills does absolutely nothing to help the body to heal. The side effects from society's rampant drug use makes us the sickest industrialized nation in the world.

Most people don't know how important their spine is. They simply think that when the pain is gone they are cured. There are many different professions that focus on people suffering from pain. General MDs, surgeons, acupuncturists, ayurveda, naturopaths, yoga instructors, homeopaths, osteopaths, and even your local neighborhood bartender can offer advice on killing pain. Why on earth as a new chiropractor would you want to join this large group of practitioners who market to and treat a limited segment of the population? I simply can't understand, from both a moral and business/marketing standpoint, why anyone would want to do this. It seems to me that it would be great to help everyone on earth reach their maximum potential. Helping people live great lives is an inspiring way to spend your time in chiropractic.

I was armed with the knowledge that the role of chiropractic, since its discovery in 1895, has never been to treat musculoskeletal conditions or any condition at all. Instead, it's a system that helps all people to live better lives. We have a system that helps all people express their lives better. Our system is an art science and philosophy that helps all people be healthier. I'm glad that from the beginning I learned that.

Chiropractors are the only professionals in the world that are highly trained to detect, analyze, and adjust vertebral subluxation. From a marketing perspective, this is good news. We're separate and distinct from any other health professional in the world. Absolutely no one else does what we do.

Do you know what percentage of the population that has vertebral subluxations? Near one hundred percent of humanity develops a vertebral subluxation at some point in their lives. The world population is rapidly approaching seven billion. We're going to need a lot of chiropractors to take care of them! This information propelled me to action. Soon all of North Georgia would know me and they too could have access to great chiropractic care.

We must begin to focus our efforts on what causes health rather than what causes disease. Chiropractic is perfectly positioned to do this. We must lead the health care transformation. We must choose to lead rather than follow other professions down the road of sickness care.

As a new student chiropractor, I knew that no matter what anyone said, I would continue to stay positive. If we want to change the level of abundance for the world's chiropractors, then we must change our focus to serving families. We must learn to serve the entire population. Instead of focusing on the ten percent of the population that suffers from neck or back pain, we must begin to focus our marketing efforts to the entire population of the planet. Imagine if dentists only focused on treating painful and diseased teeth, rather than the maintenance of healthy teeth? How would the quality of all of our lives be affected?

We need to stop acting like medical doctors. We are not medical doctors. We are chiropractors, and that is a glorious distinction! I don't know where we ever got this idea that medicine is somehow superior to us. Why do we constantly look to them for approval? Medicine is not better or worse. Medicine is different. Its objectives are different. Let's congratulate medicine for the good job that they do in crisis care and with bodies that have limitations of matter. Then let's congratulate ourselves for our ability to help people improve the quality of their lives by liberating any interference to their nervous system.

Having studied the map, my plan was to drive up to the northern clinic and then get out of the car and walk. I was going to go door to door to every business and residence to tell them the chiropractic story. To help accomplish my goal, I dressed the part and even brought props to make my presentations more fun and dynamic. In the stifling Georgia heat, I dressed in my best suit. I wore a dress shirt, slacks, tie, shoes polished and gleaming, my blue clinic jacket over my suit, and of course my pockets full of my business cards. This garb made me unusual enough to look at but then I added one thing which was sure to grab people's attention. I attached a guitar strap to each end of a plastic spine model that I had used to study spinal anatomy. Then I slung the spine across my back.

Driving the thirty minutes north on I-75 my ego begged me to turn the car around and go home to the safe and familiar surroundings of my air- conditioned condo. I "hypnotized myself" on the ride north that this was my definite purpose; this is what I had to do. I listened to an audio cassette of Dr. Sid Williams, as he motivated me to push myself to the limits of my comfort zone, and beyond. I repeated over and over as my body shook from nerves. "I can, I will, and I must... I can, I will, and I must" That mantra gave me two things: courage, and the determination that failure would not be an option.

As I got out of my poorly air-conditioned 1984 Chrysler Laser, I was immediately hit with a wall of heat and humidity from a Georgia summer in July! I almost wilted, but my mind said "I can, I will, and I must!" and my body obeyed. I walked up on to the porch of the first house and knocked on the door.

What sounded like large dogs began to bark ferociously, and in my mind I thought, "Oh great, here it comes! Killed by dogs and I just passed part three of the boards!" A little old lady came to the door with the sweetest southern drawl. She must have been shocked to see this overdressed young man with a plastic spine on her porch, but with true southern hospitality, she took everything in stride. She greeted me kindly and I went into my prepared speech.

"Hello Ma'am. My name is Liam Schübel and I am a student at the chiropractic college in Marietta. We've just opened a new clinic close by. I am going door to door to tell people in the community about the high quality low cost chiropractic care that we are offering to the public. Have you ever been adjusted?"

I was so excited that I don't think that she understood a word I said, but the ice was broken. I could do it! My strategy was to knock on forty doors a day for as many days as it took. If the answer was no, then I'd still explain with my spine how chiropractic works. If the answer was yes, then I'd ask them if I could call on them to invite them for their first appointment. Regardless of their response, before leaving I'd hand them my card, shake their hand, and thank them for allowing me to speak with them today about chiropractic.

Most responses were friendly. After all, I was on a mission to help them. My primary intention was to help people. I spoke about how to live a better life with chiropractic care. My experience has always been that the more you give, the more you receive. You can't out give the giver.

Of course, occasionally people would be rude to me but I never took it personally. After all, I was interrupting their day, I was uninvited, and in my mind, if they didn't want what I had, that was not a reflection on me. They were rejecting my offer, not me.

When someone would refuse me or ask me to leave, I'd say in my mind "next," and instantly focus on giving the best presentation ever to the next person who answered the door. I convinced myself that I was like a Good Samaritan who finds himself in a burning hotel, knocking on doors to save the people inside. If someone refuses to leave or insults you while you are trying to save their life, you just move on quickly to the next person. Having a mission many times bigger than yourself will allow you to conquer doubts, fears, and issues of low self-esteem.

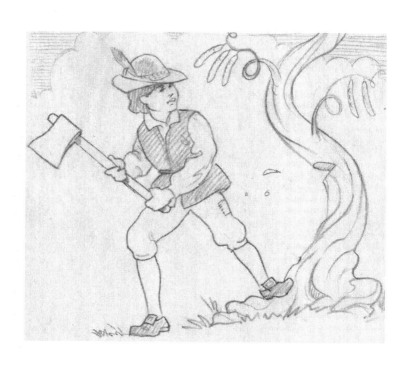

CHAPTER 8

A giant awakens

Liam

Staying positive was how I built the largest student practice in the college clinic and finished all my clinic requirements early, while others struggled but wouldn't take any advice. I have my whole life beat to a different drum, which has made all the difference. After all, a wise man once said that if you think, say, and do what everyone else does, you will tend to get what everyone else does. I didn't want to suffer and worry about meeting my clinic requirements like everyone else did. I wanted to be abundantly successful so I developed a unique plan to accomplish those goals.

I loved taking care of people in the clinic, in spite of all the medical procedures that we were required to do by the CCE. I began to see firsthand how, even with my beginner's ability to adjust subluxations, people would get incredible results. I saw chiropractic strongly impact and improve the quality of people's lives. This propelled me to learn more about the many techniques that there are in chiropractic.

I learned that the innate intelligence of the body was never to be underestimated. I learned to be thankful that the human body hadn't read the same medical books that we and the medical doctors had. I was able to witness many miracles.

There are two people that I clearly remember as a student that impacted me deeply as to just how great chiropractic and the innate intelligence of the body are. My first amazing person was Glenn. He was one of my first patients, and seeing his great response to the chiropractic adjustment was what gave me confidence in my developing abilities as a new chiropractor.

I received a phone call one day from Glenn, a mechanic who received my card from a friend. Glenn didn't walk into the clinic. He was wheeled in by his buddy, who, with a big smile, introduced us and told Glenn, "This is the guy I was telling you about."

Glenn's pain was so unbearable that he couldn't sit still, and he most definitely couldn't walk. I thought for sure that the clinic doctors were going to refer him out. He was in a cold sweat and actually shook in agony. He was dressed like a stereotypical southern mechanic, wearing an old greasy baseball cap, a Lynyrd Skynyrd tee-shirt, torn, oily, jeans, and black steel-toed, greasy work boots. He had long blonde hair. From certain angles you might have even confused him for a woman. Scraggly beard, earrings, and tattoos up and down both arms finished Glenn the Southern mechanic's dress code.

It must have been hilarious to watch from afar. Glenn and I could not have been more opposite. I think neither he nor I were happy to see each other. I was scared to death that this man's care was going to be my responsibility, and I don't think that he was too happy because he was suffering and completely miserable. At least before, he was at home in comfortable surroundings. Now he was in the hands of this newbie student intern.

I did my best to act as if I'd seen cases like his every day of the week, but I'm not a good liar. I'm positive that the only reason he stayed was because he couldn't stand up and run out! I asked him to get on the table so I could check him. This took ten incredibly long, slow, pain-filled minutes of steady pushing and pulling, until we finally got him on the table. I then began two hours of torturous and irrelevant CCE mandated exams. Even at clinic we couldn't escape bureaucracy. I didn't have the heart to tell Glenn that, because of the many rules, we weren't going to be able to see his X-rays in order to start helping him until the next day at the earliest.

I had the job of explaining all this to Glenn as I wheeled him out the front door. I promised him I'd get the paperwork done and X-rays analyzed as fast as humanly possible, and told him I'd call him when everything was ready.

The next day in the early afternoon I managed to get clearance to adjust, so I called Glenn to tell him the good news. Glenn answered in a sleepy and pain laden voice, "Yeah?"

"Hi Glenn, this is Liam Schübel from the chiropractic clinic. How are you today?"

On the other end I heard a sigh, and Glenn mumbled "not too good."

"Well Glenn, I have some good news! The X-rays are ready and we can start getting you adjusted."

"Uh, okay, what time?"

"How does 4pm sound?"

"Okay."

"Okay Glenn, see you then!"

I love the feeling that I get when I explain an X-ray to a person for the first time. The human body is so amazing, and it's a privilege that we chiropractors have to be able to share the explanation of how a person's body works with them. To see that look of interest and wonderment in a practice member's eyes is priceless. I love the fact that I can communicate the complicated aspects of the human organism in a way that is easy for anyone to understand. This skill puts people at ease and builds their confidence in our new relationship as doctor-practice member. Developing that bond is one of the fruits of our labor as chiropractors.

Glenn arrived thirty minutes early for his appointment. He had beads of sweat running down his face, and his shirt was damp from the profuse perspiration brought on by his pain and nervousness. I found out later that he was not sure if he was ever going to be able to walk again. He was afraid he was going to lose his job and his girlfriend, basically, everything that was important to him. I wish that Glenn had known that my number one priority was the same as his: helping him to be healthy again.

I wheeled him over to the view box and began to explain what I knew to be true. I was afraid for him, and afraid for me. In a way we were both about to be put to the test.

Dr. Sid Williams used to say that in the army, they teach you during basic training that when you are in a fearful state, like having bullets and bombs blowing up all around you, the way you get through it mentally is to "do what you have been trained to do."

We see many people that have been taken down a long terrible medical road. Often times, people come to see us as a last resort. What I've learned over the years is to never underestimate the body's capacity to heal when an adjustment is given and interference is removed. No matter how bleak or frightening a condition has become, I always remain calm and do what I have been trained to do as a chiropractor, and that is to adjust subluxations to restore the flow of mental impulses over the nerves.

Sometimes I hear chiropractic described as alternative medicine. That always gets me angry because it just goes to show you how medicine has become an absolute cultural authority in our society. The idea that invasive and dangerous medical drug treatments should be tried first, rather than natural conservative methods of health care like chiropractic, is absurd. Yet many people still don't have a chiropractor on their family's health care team. With less than ten percent of the population in the USA under chiropractic care, we are certainly a third world nation when it comes to taking care of its delicate and vitally important spine and nervous system.

We have to wake America up. But first we need to wake up some chiropractors. We need to speak in a unified voice that is rooted in chiropractic principles. We need to get the message out that every family needs chiropractic care.

Now back to Glenn and me in the X-ray room. As I explained his X-rays, I saw something happen to the expression on Glenn's face. For the first time he showed signs of hope rather than fear. He'd been through the mill with me for the past two days and had stuck it out from pure desperation. Now he had a look of inspiration and that inspired me as well. That change in mindset is a crucial aid to the healing process.

Now that the X-rays were explained, it was time to get Glenn adjusted. Once again, getting him in a position where I could work on his spine was an event in itself. He was in severe pain, but I finally was able to get him in a position where I could adjust his neck. That adjustment was my best! With his cervicals clear, his entire body began to relax. I was then able to get his low back adjusted.

When the adjustment was finished, I told him he was going to walk with me. He looked doubtful. He had not been able to even take one step for the last two days. I think he thought I was nuts but once again his desire to heal was tremendous. He grabbed my shoulder and I helped him straighten up. He smiled, he was up on his own two feet! He walked baby steps and in a very gingerly fashion but he was walking.

He looked at me with a look of surprise and doubt. "Is this normal?" He asked. "For you it is, Glenn. For you it is!" I left that day thanking God that I was chosen to be a chiropractor. If I had this capacity to impact this man's life with so little experience, then my future was going to be great.

I saw Glenn throughout my college career. He came in every week, and when I was leaving, I transferred him to a new student chiropractor. I've moved around a lot in my life, and it is always sad to leave practice members that you've developed a bond with. They become your extended family, and you think about them often. I wonder what ever happened to Glenn, and I hope he still gets adjusted. I hope he's found a chiropractor that loves giving care as much as I do.

Erin was another person that I had the privilege to see regain her health. She came to me with a medical diagnosis of epilepsy. She'd developed this in her late teens, and was now a college student studying business administration.

Her course work was intense, and she was under a great deal of stress.

The medical treatment for epilepsy can be brutal. It mainly consists of giving drugs that depress the nervous system. These drugs can bring about side effects and in some cases even death. Erin didn't come to me to treat her epilepsy. She came to me because she had heard that people under chiropractic care in general get great results with headaches. Erin had brutal migraines. Her migraines altered the way she lived her life and her view on the world. With the combined medication for the migraines and for epilepsy, Erin was a toxic mess. She suffered from abdominal discomfort, dizziness, and her skin was in poor condition. Good days for her were only slight sick days. Her life revolved around sickness.

After the two hour medical exam we took some X-rays for a chiropractic analysis of her spine. I made an appointment with her to go over the X-ray films the next afternoon. She had what I've found to be classic in these cases: tremendous Atlas-Axis subluxation.

It is what has been coined by B.J. Palmer in his upper cervical work as a "kink." It's where the Atlas shifts in one direction and the Axis moves in the opposite direction, coupled with very steep occipital condyles. This type of subluxation puts maximum pressure on the brain stem. It was obvious why she was so sick. I did my best to explain it all to her. She looked frightened and bewildered. Everything I said was against what she had been told for the last five years about her condition. She was completely convinced by medics that she would always be sick. I gave her my best toggle adjustment and sent her home.

The next day she came in scared. She had a seizure in the middle of the night. She described it as being different, she couldn't explain it, but she was clearly frightened. I was concerned, but I knew that in many cases symptoms sometimes get worse before they get better. I didn't want her to discontinue care, and I knew from my chiropractic analysis and pre and post leg checks that she was absolutely clear of nerve interference when she'd left the clinic.

On today's visit we needed to re-check her for subluxation. I told her that the decision would be hers alone in regards to her condition, and that she could consult with her medical doctor if she was unsure. I explained that I was here to make sure her nervous system was free from interference. She'd spent a long time on the medical carnival ride of drug therapy, and although chiropractic was frightening for her, she decided her body deserved a chance to be well.

As her care progressed during the first few weeks, she had fewer migraines but more frequency of seizures. Then on her sixth visit, I saw that her body was holding an adjustment. By my checks, she was clear. I was ecstatic! I was absolutely sure that chiropractically, we were doing the right thing.

I explained it to her, but she remained doubtful because she still felt so sick and worn out from the increased seizures. I told her to be patient. Shortly afterward, the seizures stopped! She was able to lower the dosage of the medication for the first time in over four years. Her skin began to clear up. Her migraines disappeared. Her stomach pain stopped, and her energy levels greatly improved.

She was ecstatic and could barely contain herself! She felt and looked fantastic. She'd transformed from a sickly person to a vibrant, energetic young woman. She was overjoyed that she now had a new life. I felt blessed that I had the chance to see how miraculous the body's ability to heal is. It is amazing what the body can do when it is free from interference to the nerves. It felt great to know that chiropractic care could deliver.

She was an enthusiastic patient and kept her appointment every week. She never had another seizure, and was able to get completely off all the drugs the MD put her on. When I graduated, she was there. She thanked me for all I had done for her and the big changes we had made in her life. In reality I knew it was not me who did the healing, it was her body. I was grateful to her for showing me how powerful good chiropractic care can be. It was exciting to witness the internal healing power that we each have inside of us.

The most valuable thing I learned while being a chiropractic intern at the school clinic was just how awesome it is to work with people. It is the best feeling in the world to be part of the health process. It's fantastic to see people bloom with vibrant and abundant health. Many of the rules, regulations, and senseless, mindless procedures that we must learn in CCE accredited colleges are there because they want to instill fear in us. Take the fear away, and the practice of chiropractic is all about giving, loving, and serving humanity with your unique ability to liberate lives by correcting vertebral subluxations.

I vowed that someday I'd create a place in the world where chiropractic care could flow unencumbered without all the fear, doubt and senseless procedures. In this chiropractic utopia, students, recent graduates, and even seasoned chiropractors could come and re-learn the beautiful art of giving, loving, and serving all humanity with the power of the chiropractic adjustment. This project would restore sanity to our world.

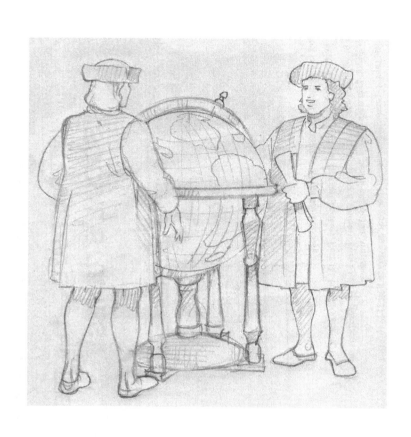

CHAPTER 9

Into the world

Judd

As a practitioner, I started with a traditional practice in a small town. How small? Four hundred families, or as we said, "Four hundred full time and more in the summer season." Why, you may ask? Frankly, I don't know why! What I needed was a good kick in the behind to tell me the obvious, which is if you want to be a great chiropractor you need to live around people.

I put in long days and sleepless nights. I did okay, but just okay. After about a year, I had a visit from my old friend Dr. Liam. Dr. Liam immediately saw the obvious, and had me act on his observations. About ten minutes later we were looking for a new location about fifty miles closer to civilization.

I reopened and put in many more long days and sleepless nights. My wife and I went house to house and door to door to each and every address in my new town of 4,000. Let me tell you, 4,000 is a whole bunch, especially when your wife is eight months pregnant in July! I expected a busy practice.

I was so excited about my first day that I arrived at the office at 5am. This was great except, by 8:45am I was like a rabid raccoon and I hadn't even seen one patient. By 9am I was ready. When the first practice member came in, I was so excited that I moved about 200 miles an hour. "Welcome! Hello! Please fill out these forms."

Adjust, and do the mini lay lecture. I didn't want to let them go. I think I walked them to the car and buckled them in so they would be safe until the next visit. That was a long day. How long? Too long! When I closed that night we had nine new practice members, and every one of them got my best, my heart and a little piece of my soul. Each one got a mini lay lecture, X-ray, and my best adjustment. I was happy, sad, worn out and energized all at the same time.

Do you know what I did the next day? I got up and did it again. I scraped and clawed like a man possessed. I put in long days and sleepless nights, giving it my all, all the time. We had open houses, pie contests, you name it. We had mailings of 10,000. We mailed our town and the towns around us. We even had a traditional sit down thanksgiving dinner for 300 people. We accepted all cases even those that could not pay. We accepted all insurances, all people, all types and guess what? Slowly we prospered.

Liam

As my life at chiropractic college began to come to a close, I began to think about plans after school. I wanted to set up practice in Florida. The thought of warm weather, beaches, and sun, combined with a growing population, made the sunshine state my goal after graduation.

Judd's grandma used to say "man plans and God laughs." God must've had a real good chuckle listening to me and my plan to move to Florida! I began to investigate the requirements to become a chiropractor in Florida, and I didn't like what I found. I'd have to work for three months as an intern for a licensed Florida chiropractor before I could sit to take the Florida Board exam.

I'm sure there are many new chiropractors that find a mentor that gives them useful information on practice. As I began interviewing with Florida chiropractors, I received some surprising offers. One chiropractor suggested I could paint his house and clean up around his office in exchange for my mentor requirements. I'd heard that some of the new female chiropractors had even worse offers. I'd jumped over a lot of hurdles to become a chiropractor, but this was one jump I was not willing to make.

I was so disappointed with the nonsense in Florida that I started to think of alternatives. One idea that became stuck in my mind was to travel and do some mission work. At the time there weren't too many opportunities to do chiropractic mission work. I became determined to travel for a while and give chiropractic care wherever I went. I kept looking for such an opportunity.

Not long after I made this my goal, my opportunity came. I walked into a class and there was a copy of the school newspaper, *Elan Vital*, on my desk. It was opened to a page that had an article about two chiropractors, Dr. Walter Sanchez and Dr. Raymond Page. They'd just opened the first chiropractic office in Peru. I read the article with growing excitement. This was it! I thought that the article on my desk was divine intervention. It was not until much later that I found out my friend Judd had read the article and figured that I would be interested so he left it on my desk!

I was impressed with the courage and dedication of these chiropractors. At the end of the article there was a Miami phone number to call for more information. I rushed home immediately and made the call. Dr. Sanchez answered the phone. I told him that I was calling to congratulate him. It was so great that they were bringing chiropractic to the world.

It shocked me when he responded with an invitation to join them. I was totally caught off guard. In my mind I had planned on doing a mission trip for a few weeks, or maybe a month tops! Dr. Sanchez was talking about a one year commitment. The more he explained, the more I liked the idea of Peru. I told Dr. Sanchez about my Florida plans, and he said, "Great, when you finish working in Peru you can do your internship in my Florida office." I accepted his offer immediately.

After I hung up the phone, I began to think about what I'd just done. Fear started to creep in. I got a sheet of paper and listed the knowns and unknowns along with the good and bad. No matter how I looked at it, it made no logical sense to move to Peru, but I just couldn't shake the inner voice that was directing me.

My final decision to go taught me to always follow your inner knower, and that your heart will always point you in the right direction. In the years since I made this decision I've come across many people who think too much. They find the negative in every situation and talk themselves out of potential opportunities because of fear. I've seen many people waste years of their life following the followers. As a result, many people never get to live up to their full potential.

The more I gave in to my inner voice, the more excited I became about the possibilities. I went to the library and took out every book I could find about Peru. What I read was not appealing. In the 1980's and early 1990's, Peru was a hotbed of social upheaval and widespread terrorism. Inflation was in the thousands of percent, and food, gas, and all basic necessities were being rationed. Poverty was rampant, and rebel groups had a stranglehold on the country. They were terrorizing the people with car bombings, kidnappings, and assassinations.

Yet, my enthusiasm would not be squelched. I chose to look at the other side of the coin: Peru was rich with a millennium culture. The ancient Incas had built civilizations unlike any in the Americas, with architecture like Machu Picchu, which to this day stumps modern day engineers with its technical and scientific specifications.

The culinary diversity of Peru is unmatched anywhere in the world. Exotic foods could be found from each of the three regions of Peru, the coast, the jungle, and the massive Andes Mountains. The people of Peru are known for their love of life, family, and fiestas. This combination of chaos and marvel attracted me. As my day to leave the U.S. became closer, I became more and more enthusiastic about this new opportunity.

Upon hearing about my latest decision to move to Peru, my parents thought I'd lost my mind, "again." My mom envisioned me as an American hostage, or worse. She put all her fear aside, however, and encouraged me to follow my heart. Much of who I am, I owe to my parents. I joke with them today that when I was young and destitute, they had to endure listening to my crazy plans. Now that I'm living the life I dreamed, they smile and tell me that they knew I would succeed because I always had so much enthusiasm.

When I told my friends and family I was moving to Peru to practice chiropractic, my mom cried, and my dad wanted to call the sanitarium and have me checked in. They're well-educated individuals, and they knew about the dangers of living in Peru during that time period. My parents have a lot of inner wisdom; there is no class that teaches you how to be a good parent. I think they must've had some divine guidance to have raised four boys, each of whom has gone on to make positive contributions to society. Thanks Mom and Dad. Words cannot express the love and devotion that I have for you.

I first flew to Florida to become acquainted with Dr. Sanchez. We spent a few delightful days in his beautiful home. Before I knew it, I found myself flying to Peru.

The airline I flew was Aeroperú. They ran some of the cheapest flights going from Miami to Lima, and they were packed with Peruvians. I think I was the only Caucasian on board. At six feet two, pale white, and a rail thin 170 pounds, with a goatee that I had shaped to look like Dr. B.J. Palmer's, I must've been quite a sight.

The flight left at around 1am and landed in Lima at about 6am. Being an overnight flight I slept my way through the night and awoke close to landing. The flight from Miami to Lima could be described as a space flight rather than an airplane flight. It's impossible to fully describe the sights, smells, and energy of the third world with words. I still find it amazing that in one day of travel, I can move from an area of extreme poverty such as exists in certain areas of Peru, to one of extreme opulence as found in many of the glamorous cities in the United States. That stark contrast is something that changes your perspective of the world. World travel allows you to get outside of yourself, and that gives you a bigger, clearer vision. I highly recommend travel to anyone.

Upon touch down, I went to collect my bags after passing through immigrations. Contained within my two well-worn suitcases, which were bursting at the seams, were all of my worldly possessions. It had taken my dad and me twenty minutes to zip them shut. After collecting my bags at the baggage claim, I groggily walked over to Peruvian Customs. The procedure is to present your customs declaration form, and if you have nothing to declare, which was true in my case, you press a button. A light then appears. Green means go, and nobody checks your luggage. Red means that Customs officials will rifle through your things looking for contraband. I pressed the button and the light turned red.

Because Peruvian sales tax approaches twenty percent, many people actually make a living traveling back and forth between the two countries purchasing cheap electronics in the USA and then selling them in Peru. I was unaware of this at the time. I thought they were checking for drugs like the customs people in the states, which shows you my naïveté at the time. Why would anyone ship illegal drugs into one of the biggest drug producing areas of the world?

After tearing my bags apart, they found nothing of interest, but they did have another problem on their hands. My suitcases had been packed so tightly that they couldn't be closed again. The customs official and I had to hold the bags together while the uniformed soldier had to lay down his machine gun and wrap duct tape around the whole suitcase. I'm sure they all still laugh about me. The funny American and his overstuffed suitcases!

Dr. Sanchez assured me that Dr. Page, who was practicing in Peru, was going to pick me up, so I wasn't worried. That was until I walked outside! At the time Peru had no organized terminal. Once you left the building to go outside you were on your own. This is where I came face to face with a throng of humanity all screaming in Spanish.

I still wasn't worried, as I trusted that any minute Dr. Page would call to me from the crowd. After all, I was not hard to spot! The minutes went by and nothing happened, then a half hour then an hour. Now I began to worry. What will I do if nobody shows up? I managed to exchange a ten dollar bill for a coin that I could use in the payphone that was probably worth ten cents. I called the only phone number that I had, which was the number of the office in Peru. The answering machine picked up and a lady's voice spoke in rapid Spanish that I couldn't understand. I wish they had saved the message that I left. It would be a great laugh to listen to it now.

"Hi, this is Dr. Schübel, I'm here at the airport waiting for someone to pick me up. Please send someone immediately! That is if you are not already on your way. Thank you!"

At this point, I thought to myself that coming to Peru may have been the biggest mistake I ever made in my life. After almost two hours of waiting at the airport, Dr. Page finally arrived. It seems that they were at a Saturday night Peruvian fiesta and had completely forgotten to come pick me up. He was in a great mood and had a disarming personality, which allowed me to quickly forget the scary experience I'd just been through.

At 9am we drove through Lima and back to the office. The first thing I noticed was that all the restaurants seemed to be packed with people, especially young people. I mentioned to Dr. Page how impressed I was that young people would get up so early on a Sunday morning just to go out to breakfast together. Dr. Page laughed and informed me that these people hadn't been to bed yet! The tradition was to come from the dance clubs which closed at 5-6am, directly to the restaurant to eat breakfast, and then go home and go to bed. Young Peruvians are nocturnal. Saturday nights last well into Sunday morning!

Arriving at the house, I went to sleep to the sounds of a Peruvian summer. People in the street outside speaking a language I was soon to learn. Ice cream peddlers were blowing a strange duck call type of whistle, letting potential clients know that the ice cream man was coming down their street. As I dozed off to sleep, I bathed in thankfulness for this opportunity that so few people on earth have the chance to experience. I'd survived an eventful twenty-four hour transfer between the first and third world, and tomorrow I'd begin my training to be the highest volume doctor in the history of Peru. Little did I know that I was a sleeping giant in more ways than one.

The people of Peru are innately in tune with natural forms of health. So naturally, they admire chiropractors and resonate with the chiropractic message. Peruvians don't trust Big Pharma. They know that much of medicine is about selling drugs, and the vast majority recognize that while those drugs can mask the symptoms, they do nothing to help the body heal.

When I first arrived in Peru, however, the grand majority of Peruvians had never heard of chiropractic. When the locals and the many taxi drivers asked me what I was doing in Peru, I did my best in broken Spanish to explain it. They gave me the strangest looks as I tried to explain. I couldn't understand why it was so confusing for them. It was not until I learned that the word quiropractica (Spanish word for chiropractic) sounded like quiromancia the way I was saying it. Quiromancia is a palm reading!

I quickly got the point that being fluent in Spanish was a necessity. My life would depend on my communication skills! Having no practice members in Peru motivated me to learn quickly. Failure was not an option, so I resorted back to the "I can, I will, and I must" attitude that had served me so well in my days at the clinic in chiropractic college.

I spent every waking hour studying Spanish. I observed Dr. Page, who was seeing hundreds of people a week. I recorded his health talk in Spanish. I then painstakingly transcribed it out, a lesson I'd learned from my good friend Judd Nogrady. I memorized his one hour presentation word for word. I memorized everything, even if I didn't quite understand what I was saying in Spanish. I even told the same jokes that he did! I was going to duplicate everything that Dr. Page did until I was busy serving people.

I once again strapped a spine on my back and went for walks in the community with my business cards. Being a giant among Peruvians, and with a very pale complexion by comparison, I must've been some sight walking down the street with a skeleton on my back! I'm still amazed to this day that nobody ever called the police on me. My guess is that in spite of the ridiculousness of my appearance, the people could feel my true intention. I had a burning desire to help.

I was on a mission to help them live their lives at their optimal potential through the power of chiropractic. Nothing was going to stop me from that goal. People are maimed, die early deaths, and suffer needlessly because they are unaware of chiropractic. Having been blessed with the knowledge of what chiropractic can do to restore optimal health to individuals is what drove me then, and what continues to drive me to this day. I live for a purpose greater than myself, and that is what helps me overcome all obstacles.

Within a month I was fluent in chiropractic Spanish. Within three months I felt comfortable traveling around by myself. As my communication skills improved, so did my practice. Within three months I was very busy. I was happy, but I wanted more. I knew I could serve more people if they only knew that I was here. There are only so many people that you can reach through one on one direct communication. Media is and always has been an excellent way to reach the masses. I decided that the next logical progression to build my practice was to start presenting the chiropractic message to the media.

I started to call around to the various radio and print media. It was no surprise that they didn't seem too interested. After all, I was a nobody to them. At twenty-seven years old, I certainly wasn't an authority in their eyes, on any subject, let alone chiropractic. I only had three months experience. What did I know?

What I knew was the power of persistence. I resolved to fax an article about a topic in chiropractic every week, and then suggested they interview me. After I sent the fax, I'd follow up with the producer of the program with a telephone call to see if he or she received it. Many refused to take my call, others were downright rude, but I persisted. I didn't take any of it personally. After all, they were only rejecting my offer, not me personally.

I was on a mission greater then myself. They were hurting their readers and listeners by not having me on. I know about the value of chiropractic, and my family and I enjoy the tremendous benefits of that knowledge. I was fighting to get chiropractic publicity for the people that I hoped to serve, not for me. It's amazing how much that attitude can drive you to take action. Dr. Sid Williams taught us to do things for the sake of doing them, to give for the sake of giving, and to love for the sake of loving. Applying this simple mindset would reap huge rewards in my life, and the lives of the people I served.

After months of constantly contacting producers, one finally called me with the opportunity to speak on the radio. I was so excited! I asked him why he'd finally decided to have me on. Was it the topic?

"No," he said, "I'm going to let you go on my program just this one time, but then you have to promise to stop calling me!" I agreed. This is where my undergraduate experience as a radio communications major finally paid off. I wasn't intimidated in front of a microphone. Screamin' Liam was about to hit the airwaves again!

As it turned out, the interview was a big success, but not for the reasons I thought. The ratings went up when I was on, so the producer actually ended up inviting me back as a regular guest. The surprise to me was why people loved to listen to me. It wasn't so much for the information that I presented, but for the enthusiastic way in which it was presented.

I sent a copy of a recording from one of my radio interviews to a friend who spoke Spanish, and asked him what he thought. His response was revealing.

"Liam, I didn't understand most of what you said, but you spoke with such authority and enthusiasm about the topic that I found myself wanting to listen to you, and wanting to come see you in your office. You clearly are motivated by the opportunity to help others through chiropractic." This is a lesson that I teach people today when I coach chiropractors. Often times it's not what you say in communication that is so powerful, but rather how you say it, and why you say it. As a result of this experience, I resolved to keep studying my Spanish until I was as authentic as a local.

I continued to work my media plan, and gradually became known as the American chiropractor who is great for ratings. It wasn't long until I was appearing regularly on radio, TV, and print media. Now the taxi drivers no longer thought that chiropractic was about palm reading. They knew it had to do with the spine, and that a healthy spine was important to a healthy life.

Being on TV is a huge ego boost. I'm not sure how many chiropractors have been asked for their autograph while eating at a restaurant, or recognized in the airport as the doctor on TV, but I do, and believe me, it's fun! My mom has even been asked if she's related to me when using her credit card while on vacation in Miami.

As B.J. Palmer used to say, "You never know how far reaching something you say think or do today will affect the lives of millions tomorrow." Television has that power, and chiropractors around the world should make it a goal to persevere enough until they too are featured on it. Our message is too important to be overshadowed by 24/7 drug ads that preach the gospel of more drugs equals better health. To stop this insanity we must all play full out, and inundate the media with the chiropractic message. Chiropractic care must become a routine part of everyone's life.

My practice continued to grow. I began to study every aspect of what I was thinking, saying, and doing in the office. I began to apply many of the principles of effective communication that I learned in my undergraduate studies to the practice of chiropractic. What I began to learn was that the better my communication, the bigger my practice grew.

When I was in school, we had a chiropractic speaker mention that when you saw 1,000 patients a week, chiropractic began to give up her secrets. I set a goal to get to 1,000 chiropractic visits a week. I'd work seven days a week, happily. I'd do whatever it took to reach my goal. I wanted to know all there was to know about chiropractic.

Many people talk about what they want or would like. I've found that commitment is one of the key factors that many people who are unsuccessful lack. Words are meaningless if they aren't backed up by persistent actions. Dr. Sid Williams used to talk about the long days and sleepless nights that are required to build a huge practice. One must surrender their self to service, and that is exactly what I did.

I was sleeping between four and five hours a day, and working seventeen to eighteen hour days. The only thing that was important to me was seeing people. I truly fell in love with chiropractic. Many people can't understand this lifestyle. It was hard work to move outside of my comfort zone, pushing the boundaries of what I thought was possible.

At this time period in my life, I never had time to feel tired. At night I couldn't sleep because I couldn't wait to get up and go to work the next day. Every day I was like a kid on the night before Christmas, excited about the opportunities that would present themselves during the course of the day.

Chiropractic practice was never boring to me. Each individual that I had the pleasure to work with was like an amazing combination lock. My job was to find the combination that would unlock the power from within them.

I learned a lot about people, communication, healing, chiropractic, love, and persistence during this time period. In the beginning of the book *Think and Grow Rich,* Napoleon Hill aptly states that the universe will give you anything that you want in this lifetime, all you have to be willing to do is ask yourself how much are you willing to sacrifice? I sacrificed my time in order to gain the mastery of the science, art, and philosophy of chiropractic. I surrendered myself to chiropractic, and the rewards have been beyond my wildest dreams.

I achieved my goal of 1,000 patient visits per week at the end of 1996. I was ecstatically happy, but I wanted more. One office was not enough to serve this country. I wanted to setup more offices, and bring more chiropractors down to show them what a wonderful life Peru had to offer. I wanted to teach a core group of principled chiropractors my system, so that they could spread out across the globe and bring about a peaceful health revolution. I wanted to create a place where chiropractic could thrive. I had a dream to create a chiropractic utopia.

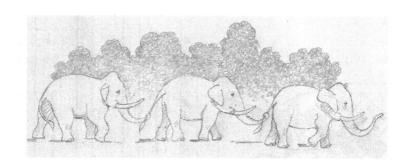

CHAPTER 10

The end is the beginning

Judd

I am in love with practicing chiropractic. Many other practitioners always talk about having a balance of chiropractic and life. I can't see how you can have a balance. Chiropractic supplies everything. We give a simple adjustment, and the principles of chiropractic supply us with everything else. I don't know how we could ever balance the equation. I don't believe we could give enough back if we lived *two* lifetimes to equal what we've been given.

When people call in the middle of the night or on a vacation day, I've always said, and will always say, I'd rather they call me than take drugs. Another thing other practitioners have always cautioned about is being friends with clients. Some of my clients have helped me with some of the greatest things in my life. My accountant has been like family. He is a client. The mechanic who fixes our cars is a client. We barter for services and I think it is the best deal in the world. If my vehicle has a problem, I call him, and within the day a loaner car arrives in the driveway and my problem is taken away to the shop. This makes me feel like a big shot every time.

I live on a farm, and I purchased it with the help of a client who knew I was looking for land. He came in one day and said, "I wouldn't tell anyone about this place except you. You've always treated me square, and I want to repay the favor, but do me a favor. If you don't buy it, please don't tell anyone else but me, because I want it if you don't." I bought the forty-five acre farm that day, and it's been heaven on earth for my family and I for the last ten years.

I can go on all day about practice members that have enriched my life beyond any monetary compensation, like the farmer that helped set up the greenhouse, the irrigation expert who put sprinklers in the greenhouse, or the excavator who helped level our fields. Being a chiropractor has put me in touch with some of the best people on earth.

In case he reads this book, I want to include the builder who built our house in ninety days, all on credit, with only a handshake as my promise to pay while we waited for the bank to finish our paperwork. And last but not least, I want to thank a man who helped me fulfill a personal dream, racing motorcycles in sanctioned races.

For a long time, all I did was adjust, with no thoughts of anything else. It was a shock to me when I finally called an accountant, and he told me how much back taxes I owed. It was no problem, I paid and kept moving. I had no clue about insurance. I just took the co-pays even if they were five dollars. I didn't care. I was adjusting people.

After about six months, one of my practice members came in and asked why I wasn't billing their insurance. I replied, "I haven't got to it yet." Many people got on my case to start billing. They said it was crazy to let all that money go.

Very reluctantly, I hired a billing lady. We were both shocked. She wanted me to start taking notes and I wanted her to just leave me alone. As we billed more, money started coming in. My accountant wanted me to become an investor. I didn't invest in anything but chiropractic. I paid off my loans and all the debt we had. We built a house, and then we paid that off.

This is a practice tip: if you want to be a successful chiropractor, strive to become debt free. It really helps in all areas of life. We're committed to a life of giving. It's a much easier to give when you don't have to worry about bills. Instead of worrying about retirement, spend your efforts on being as healthy as possible, so you can work until you're around 105.

I did my very best to practice straight chiropractic for my first two years. I practiced as a cash only chiropractor, and then insurance slowly crept into my practice. I rationalized that by accepting insurance, I was making it easier for people to get and stick with care. I rationalized that the time spent filling out forms and doing other useless insurance related activities was worth it.

Our job was to help people live better, healthier, happier lives yet we thought we could put numbers on it and call it something else. Practicing chiropractic with insurance restrictions became a huge distraction. Instead of placing my full focus on people, we were filling out forms.

One day it hit me like a Mack truck carrying a load of bricks. I was ordering party supplies for our upcoming ten year practice anniversary celebration. That day should have been my day, but it was flat. I had it all, the big practice, the big house, and all the things that everyone said were so important. Yet I knew that somehow, true chiropractic had been lost in the shuffle, and I knew that in my heart that I couldn't practice another ten years like this.

Chiropractors are supposed to be in love with service, in love with loving, and I was filling out insurance forms. I dreamed about being an old time practitioner and practicing until the day I died, but instead I was dead in practice. Do you know what I did that day? I quit! I started the process of slipping and checking. I took all the forms and paper I had accumulated and cold hard quit.

I backed up my van to the front doors of the office and loaded it up, and drove it home. Then I made a huge bonfire in the backyard, and I danced around it!

Next, I drove back down to my office. About a block away was this little store called Edeterals convenience store. I went in and bought a notepad and new pen, with which I wrote one word: "CLOSED." I stuck that note in the door, and that was that. I was out of chiropractic, or so I thought.

Now here is where being in love with chiropractic really helps. If it'd only been a passing interest, or a one night stand, it would've been over. But I really loved her, and like a true love, when you are down, she picks you up. There is no balance, no give and take. Give your heart, and she gives everything else, "that is the big idea."

Here is where it helps to have the love of chiropractic deep inside you. There was no way she was going to let me go, not with all the training of upper cervical, not with ten years of dedication to the chiropractic relationship. There was no way that was going to happen, and sure enough, my home phone began to ring.

Where was I? Where did I go? Was my family OK? All the usual pleasantries then another few weeks went by. I got calls from personal injury lawyers - I told them sorry, I was closed. I got calls from workers compensation – I told them the same thing, sorry I'm closed. I got calls from the HMO because my paper work was late – sorry, closed. A few HMO's actually tried to get me to fill out paper work to quit!

One day around 11am there was a knock at the back door. A practice member was there. This wasn't a guy that you'd ever think got the big idea about chiropractic. He never told me what a good guy I was. He wasn't particularly pleasant, nor did he come to office parties, or even acted like he cared. But there he was.

"Hello, sorry to bother you doc, but I have two problems. One, my son is sick and he needs an adjustment, and two, my lower back is killing me, and none of these jokers out here can figure out that the problem is in our necks just like you taught us. Now I hate to intrude, and I don't know why you won't come out, but we'd like to come in and get adjusted."

What could I do? Slam the door in their faces? Of course not! So I said come in, and then I was reunited with the love of service. I wish the whole dialogue was recorded, because it was so beautiful, especially the next part when his son came in, looked me up and down as only a child can, and then asked why I was in my underwear!

All the years of practicing a perfect presentation, all the years of perfecting handshakes and office policy, and here I was adjusting in my underwear!

From that instant, I knew that chiropractic was too important and too big for any one person. I knew that I had to become involved in a worldwide movement. I knew it was time for me to start connecting with other chiropractors. I was completely in love with the art, science, and philosophy of chiropractic. I had to find a way to explain to practice members, and to other chiropractors, that chiropractic is for the masses, something to be shared with everyone.

As soon as I made up my mind that I would practice again, it was as if by magic that others knew it also. I began seeing people in my garage, and then my living room. With the help of some of my people, we converted my basement into an office. As chiropractic flowed through me, I began to get offers to practice and teach chiropractic all over the world.

I started teaching a class on technique enhancement that showed other chiropractors, not how to adjust, but how to be the best in their chosen technique. It gave them a chance to understand how important attitude and clarity is in practicing chiropractic. For many, it taught them how valuable their adjustment and mindset was. Teaching the class has brought me into contact with many chiropractors, and for me that's made a huge difference. It's important and electrifying to be surrounded with like-minded people.

In the beginning, I began practicing chiropractic with the attitude that I would make my little piece of the world as safe and as healthy as possible. I believed that protecting my little corner was going to be my life's work. Chiropractic pushed me out into the world, not because that's where I wanted to go, but because that's where she wanted me to go.

All chiropractors need to let chiropractic be the love that propels them into the world, because the people of the world need us, and they need what only chiropractic can deliver, which is a chance to live the best and most abundant life possible.

We have a long and sometimes difficult road to travel, but we are humanity's last and best hope at a world of peace. Sometimes the job ahead may seem too big for you. That is when you reach out to a friend. All your dreams can be realized if you possess a willingness to learn, a willingness to let go of old thoughts and negative patterns, a willingness to love and serve, and finally, a willingness to live for something bigger than yourself by helping others.

Liam

1997 was the year that Schübel Chiropractic Centers (Centro Quiropractico Schübel) officially opened its doors. Peru was about to witness a massive transformation. The rebels had been defeated and the country began to blossom. I knew that Schübel Chiropractic would play a crucial role in serving the people in the coming years.

I am proud of the fact that I have put the term "chiropractic" into the daily lexicon of most Peruvians. When I first arrived in Peru, most of the people had never heard of chiropractic. I am prouder yet that the term chiropractic conveys an image of a chiropractor using his hands to remove vertebral subluxation from the spine. Through massive media coverage we have conveyed the chiropractic message in its pure form.

In a country with no preconceived notions about chiropractic, I was perfectly positioned to learn from the many mistakes we'd made in promoting and positioning chiropractic in the United States. I was determined to create a chiropractic Utopia. Peru would become a place where its people would "of course!" have a chiropractor. It wouldn't be a question of whether you and your family were under chiropractic care, but a question of who is your chiropractor.

It was at this point in my life that I realized why God had sent me to school to study communications. If you are going to provide a service as big as chiropractic, you better well be prepared to communicate the message to the masses. A degree in communications helped prepare me for this awesome responsibility, and my plan to make the name Schübel synonymous with pure chiropractic.

The strategies I used to build my student practice at chiropractic college were the same strategies that I used to build a booming practice in Peru. Of course, my practice in Peru grew even faster because I wasn't bogged down by the numerous restrictions and insurance issues that chiropractors in the United States have to deal with. I strapped the model of the spine to my back and began going door to door with my business cards, broken Spanish, and an unquenchable desire to liberate the planet from the ravages of vertebral subluxation.

Needless to say, the Peruvian people responded to the message. They came in droves. In three months I was seeing 500 people a week and had to expand my office hours to be able to see more. I was living in my own chiropractic heaven, but I wanted more. I wanted to increase my ability to serve. I set 1,000 visits a week as my next goal.

By now, my Spanish speaking ability was sufficient to really communicate. In the beginning, my language skills were limited and my passion and enthusiasm were what drove our success. As my language skills improved, my office exploded even more. The passion for chiropractic is what powered me in those days. I was eating, sleeping, and living pure chiropractic.

How many of us pass our days just going through the motions in our practices? We have the tendency at times to become robotic, and lose touch with the knowledge that we as chiropractors truly work with the power that animates the living universe. We've been blessed to be the only doctors in the world that are highly trained to detect, analyze and adjust vertebral subluxations. I feel it's of great importance that each and every chiropractor reminds themselves of these facts every day before they take care of the people they're so privileged to serve.

As I became better known on the radio, and my Spanish improved to a point where people could completely understand me, an opportunity to talk about chiropractic on national television occurred. I still laugh when I view those first interviews. I had a cheap 1970's suit that look like it came from a person in a mortuary who was two sizes bigger than me. I was sporting an afro and a goatee trying to emulate Dr. B.J. Palmer, while thinking that facial hair would hide my youthful inexperience. Some people said I looked like a white mix of Jimi Hendrix and Malcolm X.

Whatever my appearance, it was again the passion to get the message to the people that I believe led me to becoming the most popular health professional on Peruvian national television. I was different from the stodgy doctors with their white coats and their incomprehensible vocabulary. I spoke in a simple fashion, used analogies, and connected with people in a loving, caring manner. The result was that every time my interview aired, the ratings soared. If you know anything about television then you know that ratings drive the TV industry.

I began to experience what I call chiropractic rock star fame. I was recognized at restaurants, in the street, and at the airport. People would actually ask me for my autograph, or would ask my opinion about their personal health challenges. I must admit this was a tremendous ego boost, because I still viewed myself as the kid from Freehold, New Jersey with the big ears and value-based clothing. It was hard to imagine that I was blossoming into the face of chiropractic in South America. Even my mother was experiencing the results of having a "famous son" when she was visiting Miami, and used her credit card, only to have the Peruvian clerk ask her if she was related to the famous chiropractor Dr. Schübel!

It's easy to rest once you've attained a certain level of success. However, I make a point to remember where I came from. I believe that with every blessing from God there also comes a tremendous responsibility. Reaching my goal of 1,000 practice member visits per week in late 1996 was very satisfying, but it left me asking the question "what next"? I decided that the next logical step was to take all the lessons I'd learned in life up until this point about success, and formulate a systematic plan to share them with others.

The plan would consist of four parts:

1. Training chiropractors to be successful.

2. Getting chiropractic to the marginalized populations of the world.

3. Improving the quality of chiropractic education in the schools.

4. Developing political strategies to ensure that the practice of chiropractic would remain fun, and that all people of the world could receive its benefits.

As with any plan, it's much more effective if you work with other like-minded people to achieve your goals.

Napoleon Hill, in his book "Think and Grow Rich", describes these people as your mastermind group. In chiropractic college, Dr. Nogrady and I were a mastermind unit. In Peru, I needed to find similar individuals whose undying passion was to bring chiropractic to the world.

Once again, the chiropractic profession would provide me with more abundance in my life, and send two individuals my way, creating one of the greatest groups that chiropractic has ever known. My partnership and friendship with Dr. Michael Sontheimer and Dr. Christopher Taylor has been a blessing to me and to the rest of humanity.

Together, we began to further develop the world chiropractic plan. We began to systematize the body of knowledge that we'd acquired over the years in how to build huge practices. We created a training ground for chiropractors that would allow them to learn while they earned. We began to open chiropractic centers all over Peru and fill them with recent graduates from chiropractic school. This total immersion program has created and attracted some of the greatest chiropractors in the world today. As the word got out that we had a powerful system to open and grow large, successful chiropractic offices, we opened more chiropractic centers throughout South America.

A year ago I was approached at a New Beginnings chiropractic seminar by chiropractic visionaries Dr. Peter Morgan and Dr. Bradley Rauch. They felt drawn to the Dominican Republic, and wanted to create a chiropractic utopia there as well. In less than six months we had one office open, and in one year we had three. Our system was proving effective and easy for a new chiropractor to learn, regardless of where they were in the world.

Dr. Nick Necak began working in one of our centers in Peru, and quickly became the most successful associate that we ever had. He decided that he wanted to take chiropractic and our system to Colombia. In 2012, we will begin opening offices in Colombia. We've had several very successful Brazilian chiropractors working as associates in our Peruvian training ground. They too will be taking our system back to their home country.

Our goal is to have hundreds of offices all over the world linked with a common goal of changing humanity. Doctors from many different nations have come to our seminar to learn the "Schübel system." They in turn are bringing chiropractic to their home countries. During the next twenty years, we will expand our system to every continent in the world. I tremble when I think of how many people will benefit from chiropractic care as a result. This is what inspires me to do more. I finally found "my answer." This is what I was called to do.

The second part of our chiropractic world plan was to create mission trips. My partners Dr. Taylor and Dr. Sontheimer were given the name of the mission trip by Dr. Jeffrey Beliveau. Upon hearing our plans, he said it was going to be "the best mission trip ever." The name stuck.

There are so many things that I love about chiropractic mission trips. One is to see the miracles that occur when people who've never been exposed to chiropractic are exposed to it for the first time in their lives. We've had the privilege to serve some of the most marginalized populations on the planet. I believe mission trips are the closest thing to doing God's work.

The other thing that I find amazing is the transformation that can be witnessed in the students and doctors that participate in these mission trips. We take students who've been medically brainwashed by the CCE curriculum and we turn them into fearless, passionate chiropractors. How long does it take us to erase four years of indoctrination in a quasi-medical education? Less than four days!

Chiropractors, by nature, are hungry to help people. They just need to be shown the proper path. The first day when they arrive on the mission trip they are confused, afraid, and uncertain. The last day of the mission trip they're banging on the doors of the hospital demanding to check the spines of the poor souls that are imprisoned there.

Some of The Best Mission trips to date have taken us to the favelas (slums) of Rio de Janeiro, Brazil, the shanty towns (pueblos jovenes) of Lima, Peru, the mountain homes of Incan decedents in Cuzco, and the jungle communities of the Amazon. If you haven't yet had the experience of a mission trip, I highly recommend that you make this a priority. It will deepen the meaning in your life as a human being and as a chiropractor.

The third part of the chiropractic world plan is to participate in the education of the future generations of chiropractors on this planet. I was blessed to be asked a few years ago to be on the Board of Trustees at Sherman College by its President. Serving on the board at an institute of higher education is a huge responsibility, and a tremendous honor. Sherman College has a rich history in protecting and promoting the principles of chiropractic. They also graduate some of the finest chiropractors in the world.

To be able to directly touch the lives of the students has been one of the greatest feelings of fulfillment in my life. I encourage every doctor of chiropractic to become actively involved with a chiropractic college, to ensure that we have top quality chiropractors, so that the greatest healing art ever discovered lives on.

Being involved in politics is crucial if we wish to have continued success in our chiropractic practices and enable everyone in the world to have access to chiropractic care. Like it or not, politics has an effect on just about everything you do in life. You can worship in whatever church you wish to because of a legalized freedom of religion, you may say what you like because of a legalized freedom of speech, and you can meet politically with whatever group you choose because of the legalized freedom of peaceful assembly.

Politicians write the laws that govern our lives. We can influence how those laws are written by becoming actively involved in the process. It doesn't have to take much of your time. There are chiropractic leaders that will lead the way for you. What's crucial, however, is that you participate and support those leaders when they ask you to do something. This means devoting your time, talent, and money. It doesn't take much of each. There are so many of us that if we all did just a little, we could change the world.

As I finish this first book, I'm in the same position as when I started it. I'm sitting on a plane headed to another part of the world (this time California) to talk about one of the great loves of my life, chiropractic. I can't help but feel nostalgic about where I've come in fifteen years in chiropractic. If I had to do it all over again, the only thing I'd do differently is work even harder. There are still so many that have not had the benefit of a chiropractic adjustment.

I hope that you've enjoyed reading what we've enjoyed writing, and more importantly, I hope that you've learned some principles of success that can help you achieve the life that you deserve, no matter what your life's calling may be. Recognize that you've been given many blessings in your life. Now is the time to go share them with others. Maybe YOU were cast to be a chiropractor too.

May God always bless you from Above, Down, Inside and OUT. ADIO y ADIOS, Liam P. Schübel, D.C. and Judd Nogrady, D.C.

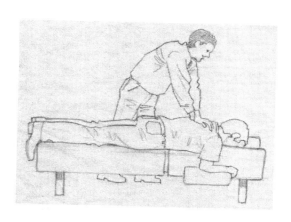

Epilogue

Currently there is regulation from the CCE that is changing many of the fundamentals taught in chiropractic colleges. These changes are taking chiropractic even further off course. There are many nationally recognized fringe groups which are trying to make the practice of chiropractic even more medical.

This is why we need you to act now! There are 10 things you can do to save this profession.

1. As a chiropractor, you need to work to be appointed to your state board. If you practice in an area of the world that does not have state boards you must become involved with whatever regulatory organization there is. We must make sure that principled chiropractic is represented. Principled chiropractors are the majority of successful practitioners in the profession but we are underrepresented in the regulatory aspects of chiropractic. We must ensure we are part of the process that keeps chiropractic laws in alignment with our views.

2. Attend your state board/regulatory board meetings – even if you are not on the board. This holds the people in charge more accountable for their actions.

3. Join a state/regional association – one that supports your subluxation centered values. If your state/region doesn't have one then start one. It is important to mastermind with like chiropractors in

your area. This will grow your practice and your influence.

4. Join the International Federation of Chiropractors and Organizations. We must start masterminding worldwide to increase our power and influence. www.ifcochiro.org

5. Support chiropractic research.

    a. Donate to these two chiropractic research organizations:

        1. Foundation for Vertebral Subluxation

www.vertebralsubluxation.health.officelive.com

        2. Australian Spinal Research Foundation

        www.spinalresearch.com.au

    b. Subscribe to a chiropractic research journal that embraces subluxation. www.vertebralsubluxationresearch.com

    c. Attend the International Research and Philosophy Symposium (IRAPS) every year at Sherman College of Chiropractic in Spartanburg, South Carolina – USA.

    Here researchers from around the world present the latest in cutting edge subluxation centered research.

    www.sherman.edu/continuing-education

6. Have a successful practice. You must live a life of abundance in order to be in a position to help the masses. There are chiropractic success seminars around the world. You need to be at them to constantly

sharpen your skills and improve your ability to serve the people of your community.

7. Join a chiropractic mission trip. Help bring pure chiropractic to a marginalized region of the world. Liberate the spark of life in an area where chiropractic has never been experienced before. www.thebestmissiontripever.com

8. Give back to a chiropractic school. You can give your time, talent, or treasure. It is time for us to pay things forward. This will ensure a bright future for chiropractic and the planet.

9. Support companies that support chiropractic. Purchase only goods and services for your practice from companies that share our desire to keep chiropractic pure.

10. Get on the media. This is one of the most powerful ways to influence the planet. It is not as hard as you think. OnPointe Seminars can show you how. www.onpointeseminars.com

We have two battles ahead, one from within our own profession, and a second with the pharmomedical* community. At this time we must create a unified force to take back principled chiropractic. We must stand together and deliver the life liberating message of chiropractic to the people of the world. Chiropractic in its essence is crucial to the transformation and evolution of our planet.

*Pharmomedical is a word coined by the author, used to describe the practice of pharmaceutical companies influencing all aspects of health care.

References

Schübel Chiropractic Training in Chiropractic Utopia

Centro Quiropractico Schübel

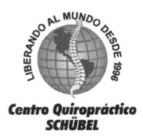

Centro Quiropráctico SCHÜBEL

www.quiropractica.com.pe

CEO – Dr. Michael Sontheimer

Opportunities now available for chiropractors and students to train and learn while they earn with us in Peru, Dominican Republic, Colombia and soon in another country near you!

We are looking for principled chiropractors that are ready to change the world! We seek associates that desire to thrive in a vertebral subluxation-centered chiropractic office, seeing high volume, being financially rewarded, learning to run a successful cash practice, learning Spanish, living/working with a team of motivated subluxation-centered chiropractors and joining the rapidly growing chiropractic movement that we are leading worldwide.

The Best Mission Trip Ever – Chiropractic Mission Trip

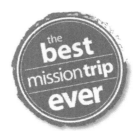

www.thebestmissiontripever.com

Co-founder and Director –
Dr. Christopher Taylor

Vision: We envision a world in which humanity lives to its optimum innate potential. A world in which individuals have the opportunity to receive subluxation-centered chiropractic care throughout their entire lives. Our envisioned world is one in which every chiropractor and chiropractic student is loving, passionate, and successful in the delivery of subluxation-centered chiropractic.

Do not miss this opportunity to travel to exotic places around the world and liberate life through the power a chiropractic adjustment. These trips will re-ignite your passion and reconnect you with your purpose on this planet!

IFCO –
International Federation
of Chiropractors
and Organizations

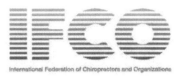

International Federation of Chiropractors and Organizations

www.ifcochiro.org

This international group is the fastest growing chiropractic organization on the planet. The top inspirational leaders and minds of the profession have assembled in this organization with one clear objective. Ensure that everyone in the world can receive chiropractic care.

If you have a vision of every man, woman, and child under chiropractic care from birth then please join and become active in helping us to liberate the potential of the planet.

The mission of the IFCO is to support and advance the practice of chiropractic that is exclusive for the location, analysis, and correction of vertebral subluxation because vertebral subluxation, in and of itself, is a detriment to the fullest expression of life. Our ultimate goal is to ensure the future of chiropractic as a separate and distinct profession to secure and insure public access to vertebral subluxation correction. We shall accomplish this by uniting and supporting chiropractors and organizations who share the IFCO mission through professional, legislative, educational and personal growth endeavors.

**New Beginnings
Chiropractic
Philosophy
Weekends**

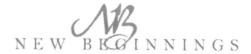 N E W B E G I N N I N G S

www.nbchiro.com

Founder – Dr. James Dubel, aka Outlaw Jim.

New Beginnings is dedicated to preserving, protecting, and perpetuating philosophically-based, principled chiropractic without compromise, innately serving mankind, while enhancing the quality of life today, creating a healthier, more perfect world.

New Beginnings is the largest gathering of principled chiropractors in the northeastern United States and is quickly becoming the international home for chiropractic's most successful leaders, worldwide.

Join the family at New Beginnings and get recharged with the newest ideas in chiropractic philosophy, success and practice management.

Dr. Schubel and Dr. Nogrady make New Beginnings their home for philosophy and principled chiropractic.

OnPointe Seminars

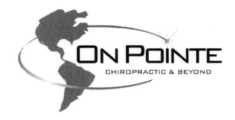

www.onpointeseminars.com

Executive Director – Dr. Liam P. Schubel

The developer of chiropractic, Dr. B.J. Palmer, once stated that the weakest link in the chiropractic profession is the chiropractic adjustment. We at OnPointe Seminars respectfully disagree. Our studies have shown that a chiropractor's ability to communicate effectively is the single most important determining factor for their success.

We have developed an entire series of powerful products and seminars that are solely aimed at improving the ability of every chiropractor on the planet to communicate the life-liberating message of chiropractic to their practice members. These communication tools have been "real world" tested in some of the largest chiropractic offices on the planet.

If you are serious about bringing chiropractic to the masses and being abundantly successful in your practice, then our products and seminars are designed specifically for you.

Hands For Change

www.handsforchange.com

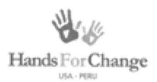

Co-founders – Drs. Chris Taylor, Michael Sontheimer and Liam Schubel

The mission of Hands for Change is to improve and empower the lives of Peruvian children through education. The company sells unique handmade finger puppets from Peru and donates a portion of the proceeds to educational programs geared towards children in the most impoverished areas.

This company also provides a steady source of income for the children's families through the production of these handicrafts. Many organizations around the world, like The Best Mission Trip Ever, World Congress of Chiropractic Students and other chiropractic clubs have used Hands For Change products as fundraisers that "give twice," allowing their organization to raise funds for both themselves and the children of Peru, thus providing a way to change the world through win-win, self-sustaining partnerships.

Chiropractic Schools - References

Check out these schools if you or someone you know may be cast to be a chiropractor.

Sherman College of Chiropractic
Spartanburg, South Carolina, USA
www.sherman.edu
Dr. Schübel is a proud member of the Board of Trustees and a Regent of Sherman College.

Life West Chiropractic College
Hayward, California, USA
www.lifewest.edu
Dr. Schübel is a proud member of the Presidents Circle at Life West.

New Zealand College of Chiropractic
Auckland, New Zealand
Dr. Schübel is a proud donor to the NZCC.
www.chiropractic.ac.nz

Barcelona Chiropractic College
Barcelona, Spain
www.bcchiropractic.es/eng/english.htm

Life University
Marietta, Georgia, USA
www.life.edu
Dr. Schübel is a proud alumni and extension faculty member at Life University.

Dr. Liam Schübel

Dr. Liam Schübel is a World Chiropractic Ambassador. He is a master of taking the chiropractic message to the mass media. He has been seen and heard by millions internationally via radio and television.

Less than a year after graduating Chiropractic College in 1995 his practice grew to 1000 visits per week. Currently he owns 14 offices in Peru and 3 in the Dominican Republic. He Co-founded a chiropractic mission trip experience like none other appropriately named www.thebestmissiontripever.com in order to help doctors and students alike reconnect with their passion to serve the masses who so desperately need what chiropractic care has to offer.

He speaks to thousands of students and doctors around the world teaching the most powerful methods to communicate chiropractic to the masses. This lead him to Co-found one of the most successful chiropractic communications companies in the world named OnPointe Seminars www.onpointeseminars.com.

Dr. Schübel serves on the Board of Trustees for Sherman College of Chiropractic and is an active member of the International Federation of Chiropractors and Organizations whose goal is to bring subluxation Centered Chiropractic to the world. Dr. Schübel is a regular speaker at chiropractic seminars like New Beginnings, the IFCO Global Summit, Cal Jam, Chiropractic Connect, Life West Wave, DE, CORE, and EPOC.

His home base is in his hometown of Freehold, NJ, where he resides with his wife Parinda and his son and daughter, Liam Jr. and Maryanne. "The Schübelnator" as he is affectionately known by on the international speaking circuit is unstoppable when it comes to bringing principled chiropractic to the world.

Dr. Judd Nogrady

Dr. Nogrady was drawn to chiropractic out of a desire to help people experience the miracle of healing with chiropractic care which he experienced personally. He graduated from Chiropractic college in 1995. He has had offices in Maybrook, NY, and New York City.

He now sees practice members at a home practice in Montgomery, NY, and does house calls. He travels internationally regularly to adjust infants and children. He is dedicated to getting the world's population to understand the vital importance of checking all newborns for subluxation.

Made in the USA
Charleston, SC
15 May 2012